Untold Stories of a
PARAMEDIC

True Stories of Life on the Job

LUCIANO NISI

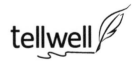

Tellwell Talent
www.tellwell.ca

ISBN
978-0-2288-0151-1 (Hardcover)
978-0-2288-0150-4 (Paperback)
978-0-2288-0152-8 (eBook)

Dedication

This book is dedicated to all the paramedics who lost their lives on the job, either from an unfortunate accident or took their own life from the effects of a psychological trauma such as PTSD.

Acknowledgements

I would like to firstly thank all my colleagues who I worked with over the years. Some of you are a part of the stories contained in the pages of this book. Many of you who knew I was writing this book provided words of encouragement and enthusiasm which helped drive me forward to the completion of this book.

To my mom, for always believing in me, and supporting me in all the things I do.

To my kids, Luke and Sierra, for putting up with your dad's constant stories and escapades which, at times, were almost unbelievable. Your happy, smiling faces and laughter remind me why I needed to tell these stories.

To all the unnamed people who, through conversation, found out I was writing this book and told me they look forward to reading it. This unilateral reminder would encourage me to write another story when at times I felt depleted.

To my editor Lee Blanding for your continued diligence in multiple revisions until the finished product.

Disclaimer

While the stories in this book are all based on real incidents, the author has changed all identifying information, omitted parts of some incidents and combined incidents for dramatic purposes. All names, places, dates, times, even ambulance call signs have been changed. Any similarity to any particular emergency incident is purely coincidental.

The medical information is accurate to the best of the author's knowledge but the author is not a physician and not qualified to give medical advice of any kind. If you have a medical condition similar to one mentioned in this book, consult your doctor.

The opinions in this book are those of the author alone and not necessarily those of the BC Emergency Health Services or the BC Ambulance Service.

Any errors in the book are, of course, solely the author's responsibility.

PTSD and OSI

An operational stress injury (OSI) is any persistent psychological difficulty resulting from operational duties performed while serving in the Canadian Armed Forces or as a member of the Royal Canadian Mounted Police. It is used to describe a broad range of problems which include diagnosed psychiatric conditions such as anxiety disorders, depression, and post-traumatic stress disorder (PTSD) as well as other conditions that may be less severe, but still interfere with daily functioning.[1]

> **Medical Definition of post-traumatic stress disorder**
> a psychological reaction that occurs after experiencing a highly stressing event (as wartime combat, physical violence, or a natural disaster) outside the range of normal human experience and that is usually characterized by depression, anxiety, flashbacks, recurrent nightmares, and avoidance of reminders of the event—abbreviation *PTSD*; called also *delayed-stress disorder, delayed-stress syndrome, post-traumatic stress syndrome*; compare combat fatigue
>
> **Merriam Webster dictionary:** Online

---

1   http://www.veterans.gc.ca/eng/services/health/mental-health/
    understanding-mental-health

'PTSD' is a group of letters that mean more to some than others. From higher levels of media coverage over the last few years, those letters are becoming more well-known, or at least what that acronym stands for. For anyone who does not have the condition or has not been involved with it, the understanding of PTSD may be fractured, and there may only be a minimal understanding as to what it means beyond the letters.

The definition of an OSI was taken from the Veterans Affairs website, though it is certainly not limited to the military or RCMP. All first responders can be affected, including paramedics, firefighters and other front line first responders. It does not include persons who sustain PTSD from other acts of violence, such as surviving an aircraft crash, sexual abuse, or other events that may cause a person to have a diagnosis of PTSD. It is intended for those whose job is to respond and deal with events often daily that cause an OSI condition.

I have met a number of people who have PTSD. Some are veterans that I served with in the military; others are paramedics, firefighters or police officers. One thing I have noticed is that although the signs and symptoms listed may occur, every individual experience it differently. Even if two people are exposed to the same event at the same time, how each of their brains processes the event will be different. There are some common trends in behavior and there are often triggers that will remind the person of an event, often in vivid detail.

I will not claim to know all about PTSD; I am not an expert and have no formal training in how to evaluate or access anyone who has it. I do have a personal close connection to the meaning though. I was diagnosed with PTSD by Veterans Affairs Canada in the fall of 2015 after an exposure while serving as a medic in Rwanda, Africa in 1994 with the Regular Armed Forces. I lived with it for 21 years and didn't know I had it. The main thing I found was I was in denial and accepting the diagnosis was a very difficult thing to accept. I felt weak, and that I should have been stronger and not let it affect me. But it did affect me. It affected my relationships with family, friends, and my marriage. I had to accept and understand that I was not broken. I had to be told multiple times by psychologists that how it affected me was completely normal, given what I had been exposed to and experienced. The part that I did not understand was that after my release from the military in 1996, when I went on to work in the Coast Guard and, later, during my career as a paramedic, I was exposed to and had to deal with many events from dead bodies floating in the ocean, to traumatic violent calls, to overdoes, to multiple cardiac arrests, often on a weekly or daily basis. I never had an OSI or PTSD effect from those calls, so I would ask myself 'Why did the event that happened in Rwanda Africa affect me?' Through my treatment, the meaning of that would reveal itself. I do understand that, at least for me, there is no 100% cure for PTSD, but rather an understanding and managing of a condition. Diagnosis and later acceptance were the biggest steps to moving forward and not letting a psychological exposure overtake my life.

Foreword

Untold Stories of a Paramedic is a compilation of real stories of calls I was involved with while working as a paramedic, mostly while working on a BLS ambulance. In all the stories, I was either the driver or attendant. The locations, towns, streets, and anyone's personal information is fictitious. The patients' age, gender, and ethnic origin do, however, represent the actual patient. The only name that is accurate is my own. At times, during an entire block of four shifts, we may never use any medications from our medical kit, or even apply oxygen. Some shifts we never use our cot and all our patients can walk easily to the Ambulance. I wanted to provide a variety of stories, including the worst calls, as well as the ugly calls. Without knowing the actual stats, I would say only 10% of our calls are of a serious nature requiring immediate life-saving interventions. In the others, some patients do need to see a physician, some could have gone to a clinic with a family member; others, perhaps, do need to go to the ER in a hospital, but their injuries are not life-threatening in nature. We also do routine inter-hospital transfers when our transfer fleet is over-booked or Emergency transfers that require a RN and sometimes a RT to attend, with the patient on a ventilator, and with multiple IVs running with various medications; these are very sick patients and these transfers are considered stat and we drive Code 3.

In the end, this book would never have been completed, as every day I go to work new stories could have been added, so I had to decide on what stories I wanted to share and how many. I hope you enjoy my personal insight into my world as seen through my eyes. Stories I have included are only a glimpse of the calls I have been on. I have included perhaps some of the more interesting or exciting calls, as they seem to stick in the memory. The truth is many of the calls we do are very mundane; indeed, many times we truly feel like a taxi service. Sometimes we show up to residences with three cars in the driveway after driving Code 3, finding a patient who does not require any immediate interventions or treatment by us, or could have easily been driven to a local clinic by the family. This patient then walks to the Ambulance, and, upon arriving at the hospital, walks to the triage area for assessment. From our perspective as paramedics we feel devalued, as there are sick and injured people who do require our care and that is exactly why we became paramedics in the first place — not to drive people to the hospital that are ambulatory. Unfortunately, the public perceives that they will get in faster if they call an ambulance; this is not the case, but it would take years of public education to change that perception. This is my first book on this type of subject and hopefully I have been able to paint a reasonable picture of what it is like to be a paramedic in BC.

Table of Contents

Glossary of terms 201

What is the process to become a Paramedic in BC? 211

Life around the station. 217

Stories from around the station 219

About the Author 229

The stories

Stab yourself

Another busy day. We were a three-person crew that day, as I was precepting a paramedic student. We had just arrived at a cross-cover location. My partner and the student had stepped away from the Ambulance with their portable radios. I settled back in my seat and closed my eyes, enjoying the quite time; our dispatch radio was turned down to low. The sun was shining and it was a very nice day...too nice to be working. I was less than five minutes into my break and suddenly the CAD sounded: "Blip...blip...blip."

I looked at the CAD, acknowledged the call, and read the information:

- Code 3 for psychiatric patient
- violent weapons, serious hemorrhage
- police on scene – scene safe."

Dispatch: "82A2[2] portable."
My partner replied: "82A2."
The CAD read "Code 3."
My partner replied: "10-4."

As I waited for them to get back to the Amb, I inputted the information in the GPS and looked up the call on the CAD mapping system. The CAD sounded again: "Blip...blip...blip."

The CAD read:

- Man, with knife cutting wrists
- Very deep cuts to wrist
- Pt stabbing himself in chest and abdomen

---

2   Pronounced: "eight-two alpha two"

I looked at the distance to the call and we were very far away – over twenty minutes, driving Code 3. I could not believe we were the closest car.

My partner arrived back at the Amb with the student and asked, "What do we have?"

I replied: "Code 3 for a psych patient cutting writs and stabbing self in chest and abdomen."

She looked at me, surprised, as she turned to look at CAD information on the screen. With a bewildered look on her face she started the car and activated the emergency lights and siren. The student in the back was excited to hear we had such a traumatic call. Students want to be faced with traumatic calls to have firsthand experience, especially under the supervision of a preceptor, so they don't have to worry about making the wrong decisions.

We headed to the call; traffic was heavy as my partner navigated through the intersections. When we finally arrived scene, there were four police cars and a fire truck on scene. I looked to my left and in a parking lot could see firefighters performing CPR on a person. There was one police officer who was placing yellow flagging tape around the scene. We got out, I grabbed the kit and suction, my partner grabbed the O2, and we headed beyond the yellow flagging tape. As I approached, I saw a Caucasian male laying on the pavement with blood all over his chest. His left arm was so badly cut it looked like someone had taken a chainsaw to it. The firefighters were doing CPR and I instructed my student to take over BVM.

I grabbed the mike on my portable radio and called Dispatch: "82A2 portable."

Dispatch: "82A2."

I responded: "82A2. CPR in progress. Multiple stab wounds to chest. Send ALS Code 3."

Dispatch: "10-4."

I approached the Fire Captain and asked him "How long have you been doing CPR?" He replied: "15 minutes with no shocks."

"Did you update our dispatch that you were doing CPR?" I asked.

He replied: "Yes we did, twice!"

"Great," I said. "We were never updated of this information."

I took a survey of the scene. There was a jeep parked inside the yellow tape line. A police officer was speaking to a woman. I looked back over at the patient, as they performed CPR. Blood was being squished out of the multiple stab wounds in the chest and abdomen. I began counting the stab wounds: there were eight. From what I could tell, the entire forearm was partially shredded off. My partner, the student, and the fire crews were performing CPR, so there was not much for me to do at that moment and, from looking at the wounds, seemed futile anyway. I was going to call an emergency physician and ask for a discontinue order but decided to wait for the ALS car, as I knew the ALS paramedic working that day. I could hear the siren of the other Ambulance approaching.

22A1 arrived and the ALS paramedic, Jon, walked up to me.

"Hey Luc," Jon said, "how long has he been down?"

I looked at my watch and did a mental calculation: "About 20 plus minutes since the first CPR was performed. The police started it and then Fire continued. This whole call is a complete screw up. We came from the bridge on cross coverage...took us over twenty minutes Code 3."

Jon said: "What?"

I replied: "Yes, we need to do a call review. We could not be the closest BLS car...and this should have been an ALS call from the beginning."

Jon said: "Yeah...we have been in quarters for the past forty minutes."

I replied: "Great...six minutes away from this call. Well, would not have mattered anyway. This guy would probably have died in the ER if he did this outside their doors. I would have called it but wanted you to attend and make the call; this is such a shit show."

"Glad you did," Jon said. "Hey, going to just check on the guys." He walked over to everyone working on the man, as I walked over to the RCMP Sergeant. "Hi, where is the knife or weapon that he used?"

The Sergeant replied: "It's in the trunk, do you want to see it?"

"Yes please," I replied. We walked over to the back of the police car and he opened the trunk. Inside in a clear plastic bag was an eight-inch long butcher knife covered in blood. I began processing that this guy had first almost sawed off his wrist, then purposefully stabbed himself in the chest and abdomen eight times...unbelievable!

I walked back to where everyone was working on the patient. Jon walked over to me.

Jon said: "Hey, do you mind if they practice a bit on this guy?...You have a student and so do I. He is long past survivability on this."

I replied: "No, not at all."

Jon said: "OK cool, I will call the doctor and discontinue in about another ten minutes or so."

"Sounds good."

I looked over to my right and noticed a woman with long black wavy hair standing next to her jeep, with a police officer; the woman seemed very upset. I walked over, and as I got closer I realized I knew the woman. I approached her and called out her name...I could see the despair in her eyes. I gave her a big hug and asked what was going on. I was told she had been the first on the scene and had begun CPR prior to the police arriving. I could not believe she had been exposed to such a traumatic scene. This was the worst stabbing I had seen since being a paramedic. We chatted a bit about counselling and I made sure I had her contact number for follow-up.

I went back to the scene where Jon was standing. Jon said: "I'm going to call the Doc and ask to discontinue."

I replied: "Good idea."

Jon made the call then walked over to everyone working on the man. Suddenly, the flurry of activity stopped. I looked down at the body... the knife wounds weeping blood from the chest cavity that was most certainly full of blood. He was no longer a patient: he was now a dead body, laying there, lifeless.

We proceeded to tie off IV lines, remove non-essential equipment and clean up the scene. Certain medical items must remain on the body as they were during the resuscitation attempts for the coroner and if there is an autopsy.

My partner and the student headed back to the car. I began to write up the call on my form, making detailed notes of our involvement in the resuscitation attempts.

We were all in the car: my partner in the driver's seat, the student in the back, writing up her student log to be signed off my me. We chatted about the call briefly, reflecting on how consuming it was and visually gruesome.

When I was done, I got out and handed a copy of my patient care report to the RCMP member. I got back in the car and my partner turned to me and said: "Time for a coffee?"

I replied: "Oh...yeah think we deserve a few minutes to unwind from this call. I'm not going to clear us until we get our coffees. Dispatch does not care what kind of a call we just did. If we clear they will give us another call...we need a few minutes."

My partner replied: "Yes, totally!"

Ferocious Animal Attack

It was another busy day. We had just cleared an MVA with no injuries and the radio squawked.

"8C1[3]"

"8C1", I replied on the radio.

"8C1 - you have a Code 3 call a few blocks from where you are. It's for a ferocious animal attack, nature of injuries unknown. You will see a car with its four-way flashers on."

"8C1 – 10-4," I replied.

Turning to my partner, I said: "Hey I wonder what type of ferocious animal attack we have this time!"

My partner replied: "Yeah, like last time I remember responding Code 3 and it was for a minor dog bite."

---

3   Pronounced: "eight charlie one"

I turned on the emergency lights and sirens and proceeded to the call. Traffic was heavy as I navigated to the call. On approach, I noticed a two-door mid-sized car on the opposite side of the street. I crossed the road and parked directly in front of the car, leaving my emergency lights activated.

As soon as I stopped, a Caucasian man approximately aged 55 (he looked European) approached my driver's side door, I rolled down the window and he proceeded to tell me his wife was viciously attacked by a ferocious animal.

My partner and I exited the Ambulance. I asked the man why type of animal it was, and he began to feverishly look at his phone, apparently looking for a photo of the ferocious animal.

At the same time his wife, a heavy-set Caucasian woman (she also looked European), walked up from beside the car...and since I couldn't see any obvious blood or wounds I became a bit puzzled. The woman very excitedly began shouting that this wild ferocious animal viciously attacked her without being provoked. I asked the woman to show me where she was bitten, my partner standing beside me now. The woman began excitedly pointing her index finger all about. I again asked where the wound was. The woman quickly and abruptly moved her left hand toward me with her index finger extended upward.

"Here!" she exclaimed. "This is where I was bitten!!"

I looked at her finger and again said "Where were you bitten?"

She pointed to the tip of her index finger now: "Here, right here!"

I took a closer look and noticed a very fine scratch at the end of her finger. There was a very fine line where there might have been a bit of blood weeping through, but I could not be sure.

"That scratch?" I asked.

She jumped back and began shouting, "Scratch!!...He bit me! I need a rabies shot immediately!! You need to give me a shot!"

My partner walked the woman to the back of the Ambulance and took her inside for some minor wound cleansing. The man, still looking for the photo, became very impatient. "I know it's here someplace."

"Well, do you remember why type of animal it was?" I asked.

He replied: "No, but it's here someplace...just have to find the photo."

A few minutes later, the back doors of the Ambulance burst open and the woman came out in a fit, shouting and screeching that we must take her to the hospital with lights and sirens going before she died."

Just at that moment the man bounded toward me in excitement and said, "This is the ferocious animal that bit her!"

I looked at the photo and saw the cutest squirrel being fed a peanut from someone's hand. The squirrel was looking rather timid as it was about to take the peanut. With a bewildered look on my face I said, "The squirrel?"

The man said "Yes, that is the ferocious animal!! It bit my wife on the finger!"

I had to look away at that moment or I would have burst out laughing right in front of them both...it was too much. 'We drove Code 3 for this?!' I thought.

I began to explain to them that we were not going to drive "lights and sirens" to a hospital that was only six blocks away, and, in fact, if they chose, they could drive up to the ER for the shot themselves, as it was not an emergency that required an ambulance.

The woman was shocked! She was beside herself. She began to quiver in disbelief that we would not drive her, with lights and sirens, to the hospital. My partner explained that we could transport her to the hospital, but not "lights and sirens."

The man and woman, frustrated, declined and began walking back to their car. My partner walked after them and had them sign our form for medical release of responsibility.

We got back into our Ambulance and drove a few blocks away, so my partner could write up the patient contact form.

"8C1" I radioed to Dispatch.

"8C1," Dispatch replied.

"8C1 – We are 10-8 Clear, patient is making their own way to the hospital."

"8C1...10-4."

As we drove away I asked my partner, "What happened?"

She said: "The woman freaked out that I would not give her a rabies shot immediately. When I explained that we did not carry rabies shots she just got up and burst through the back doors to get out."

I began laughing so hard now I could barely see to drive, thinking of the whole chain of events.

"I almost split a gut laughing when he showed me that photo of that cute squirrel," I said. "It was too funny! And her wound...it was a scratch!"

Laughing, my partner said "Yes, no kidding...unbelievable!"

Tooth Extraction

It was a very busy night in the city, non-stop since we started. We had just returned to our station. It was 2:00 am, and I was looking forward to a bit of downtime, maybe even an hour to relax our minds from the non-stop calls, grab a bite of food, and unwind for a few minutes. Earlier this evening we had attended a stabbing. We had just walked up stairs and sat down when the hotline rang!

My partner 'Doug' sighed: "No way...already? Geez we just got back...now what?"

I replied: "I know, right? We just got back. Wonder what 'emergency' there is now?"

Doug answered the phone: "17A2."

I could hear Doug say: "Really...you are kidding!?"

He hung up the phone and said: "You won't be believe this...seriously you won't believe it!"

"What?...What is it?" I asked.

"We are going to a toothache...." There was a pause of silence in the room as I processed what Doug said.

I replied: "A toothache...seriously? At 2:15 in the morning? Wow."

We headed down to the car. Doug grabbed the radio mike: "17A2."

Dispatch: "17A2."

Doug: "17A2...you can show us 10-8."

Dispatch: "10-4."

Doug was driving tonight. I waited until we almost pulled up to the call to write up the call as often we are diverted to a higher priority 'Code 3' call. I handed Doug the patient care form and went to the side door to grab the jump bag.

As we headed into the call, I noticed an opened door as we approached. There was a slim Caucasian man in his 40s standing at the door. He motioned for us to come inside.

Doug said to the man: "Are we here for you?"

The man replied: "No, my roommate...he is upstairs."

We followed the man upstairs. The condition of the house was untidy, but not as bad as I had seen on other calls. When we reached the top of the stairs we entered the living room and a Caucasian man in his 40s was sitting on the couch.

I put down my jump bag and approached the man.

I said: "Hi...are we here to see you?" The man (now our patient) replied: "Yes."

I replied: "What can we do for you tonight?"

The patient replied: "I have a toothache, and it's killing me I can't stand it any longer."

"OK...how long has this been bothering you?"

"Well...about two weeks now."

I paused as I processed what he had told me: that he had called 911 at 2:00 in the morning for an ambulance...for a tooth ache.

I replied: "Well, have you seen a dentist?"

The patient replied: "No...I was hoping the pain would go away... but it didn't."

I replied: "Well what has made it worse this evening that you would call an ambulance at 2 am from over a week ago when it started to hurt?"

The patient replied: "It's just...I can't take the pain anymore."

And with a straight face I replied to him: "Do you have a pair of pliers?" As I said this, I turned to the roommate for confirmation that they had pliers in the house. I glanced at my partner who had been recording the man's personal information (name health #, DOB etc.), and a subtle smile came across his face.

The patient, looking rather confused at my question said: "Yes...I believe we do."

"Great!" I replied "...Can your roommate go grab them please?" I looked over at the roommate as if to indicate that he go retrieve the pliers.

I said to the roommate: "Can you grab the pliers for me please?" The roommate, looking rather confused, left the room.

The patient, looking rather anxious as he grabbed his jaw said: "What do you want with the pliers?"

Just then the roommate returned with a pair of split-lock plumbers pliers and said: "Will these do?" I looked over at him and the pliers. I motioned for him to hand them to me, he did, and I looked them over and said: "Yes, I think these will work."

The roommate, looking even more puzzled than before, just stood there.

The patient, looking extremely anxious now, repeated what he had said: "What do you want with the pliers...what are you going to do with them?"

I looked over at him and, in a very calm demeanour, slowly moved in toward the patient (a few feet away now) and replied: "Well...I'm going to extract your tooth for you of course!"

The look on the patient's face was that of horror and disbelief! He replied: "No you're not!...What?"

I replied: "Well, I have about as much training as an emergency room physician in tooth extraction, so we might as well save you the trip."

Continuing, I said: "Do you know why dentists become dentists?"

The patient replied: "Uh...no."

I replied: "Because they don't have to be up at 2:30 in the morning!! Look, we will gladly take you to the emergency. You will sit there for about four hours, and they might give you some Tylenol 3s, then send you home and tell you to see a dentist...your choice."

The man looked a bit bewildered now...still holding his jaw.

I said: "Do you have any Tylenol or Ibuprofen here?"

The patient replied: "Uh...we might have some."

I replied: "OK well either you come with us or you can take some over-the-counter medication as long as you are not allergic or have any sensitivities to it...I cannot advise you on what to take or what to do — it is your choice. I am just giving you the facts of what is probably going to happen if we take you in. So, what would you like to do?"

The patient replied: "Uh...well, if they are not going to really do anything then I might as well just not go and see a dentist tomorrow."

I replied: "Excellent idea...are you sure though? We will take you right now if you want to go."

The patient replied: "No, I don't want to wait four hours for Tylenol."

I replied: "OK, I will just get you to sign my patient care form, stating that you refused transportation and treatment to medical care."

The patient signed my form, witnessed by his roommate. I advised him that he could call us back at any time and we left the house.

When we got back into the car, my partner started laughing uncontrollably. "I can't believe you did that!" Doug said, laughing. "I had to do everything but burst out laughing when the roommate came back with the pliers and you moved in toward him."

I replied: "Well...really? He calls an ambulance for a toothache? I couldn't resist."

Doug replied: "Well never seen anyone do that...too funny." He grabbed the radio mike and said: "17A2."

Dispatch responded: "17A2."

Doug replied: "17A2 we are 10-8 clear patient refused AMA (against medical advice)."

Dispatch: "10-4" — we could hear a laugh in his voice — "you are clear for home."

Doug replied: "10-4."

Doug drove back to the station and we ended up getting a couple hours of downtime. What a night.

Headshot

The shift was half way over. We had done a few calls, but nothing serious. I had never worked with this partner before and we were just chatting about calls we never go to as we proceeded to 'cross-cover' another community. (When ambulances are not available in a nearby community, an ambulance is sent to sit in between both towns.) I was driving this shift, traffic was light, and it was night now.

"Hey, what calls have you done?" I asked my new partner.

Sue replied: "Well I have done a lot of variety, I guess, but never done a shooting."

I replied: "Funny you say that. In nine years I have never done one either — a few stabbings, but never a shooting. Kind of odd actually. Figure I would have gotten a call to attend one day in all those years."

Sue replied "Yeah, actually I have not done very many serious calls, never even a stabbing."

Just then the CAD went "Blip...blip...blip" (the sound indicating a call was coming in). Sue turned the CAD and looked at the screen. "You won't believe this...we are going to a shooting! Man was shot in the head, we are the closest car."

I replied: "No way! You're kidding, right?"

Just then the radio squawked: "23A2."

I picked up the microphone and responded: "23 Alpha 2."

Dispatch: "23A2 – we are sending 75A1 (Advanced Life Support Ambulance). They are 15 min away. We are also initiating auto-launch (an air ambulance was being dispatched to the call). Fire Department is en route; police are at the scene."

"10-4," I replied.

I activated the emergency equipment and the siren began to wail as I drove...a bit faster than I normally would. I could feel an adrenaline rush through my body as I thought of all the possibilities.

The traffic was light on the rural two-lane road as I proceeded to the call.

As we approached a very well-lit intersection, we could see four police cars and a fire truck. A car was sitting part way up a meridian to the four-lane roadway. Police tape ('Do Not Cross Police Line') had already been taped away from the scene across the police cars that were keeping people away. It was late at night and the streets were bare of people and traffic.

As I approached, one of the police officers opened the tape and we drove right up to the car on the median. I stopped the Ambulance and clicked the "on scene" button on the CAD. I could see three or four firefighters on the side of the car and a body lying on the street a few feet away from the car. Sue and I got out of the Ambulance. I raced around the back of the Ambulance and grabbed the suction and the O2 (oxygen tank) and proceeded to the scene; Sue had already grabbed the jump-bag (our pelican case with all our equipment and drugs).

As I approached, I could see the firefighters hovering around the man on the ground. He was not moving.

Sue started to freak out! "Why are you not doing CPR?" She shouted to me: "We need the BVM (Bag Valve Mask), and the AED (Automated Deliberator). Sue exposed the chest and began chest compressions.

A little confused, I asked the firefighters: "Why didn't you guys start CPR?"

A firefighter replied: "He was shot in the head. There is a bullet wound right here." He pointed to the entry wound of what looked like a medium calibre round.

I looked for an exit wound, but there was none.

Sue screeched again "Get the AED!!" This is not obvious death!" I instructed the firefighters to take over CPR as I rushed to the Ambulance side door and grabbed the AED.

Sue assembled the BVM and began ventilating the patient. I applied the pad of the AED and turned the unit on. As I turned it on, it made a "doooooodit blimp" sound, and an artificial voice announced: "Press analyze."

I pressed the 'analyze' button and the voice said: "Stand clear! Stop CPR." I shouted: "Stand clear, everyone stand clear!" Everyone moved away from the patient. The AED announced: "Stand clear, analyzing now" (The AED was analyzing for a shockable arrhythmia). The AED announced: "No shock advised continue with CPR." I shouted: "Resume CPR!"

I got up now and began looking inside the car for a firearm. As I did, I noticed what looked like a .38 calibre revolver on the floor of the car, and as I scanned the car I noticed bits of brain matter on the passenger seat. It was clear to me that this man had shot himself in the head.

I asked the firefighters: "Was he out of the car when you arrived?" A firefighter replied: "No he was in the car and we pulled him out onto the street."

I looked over as Ambulance 75A1 pulled up. CPR was still in progress. The ALS crew approached and began taking over the treatment of the patient.

As a group, we loaded the patient onto a Clamshell (or ROS, for 'Robertson Orthopaedic Stretcher') a device that splits in two and is placed underneath a patient to lift them from the ground onto a cot or extricate them from an area.

The patient was loaded in back of the Ambulance and treatment continued, including CPR and bagging (BVM). Two large-bore IVs were initiated, and advanced drugs were given: Atropine, Epinephrine, Sodium Bicarbonate, and a few others. The patient was intubated (tube placed down the throat with air balloons on the end).

We drove to a nearby school where an air ambulance (helicopter) was waiting for us. By this point, we had gotten his pulse back and were no longer doing CPR. The patient was loaded onto the helicopter and flown to a nearby trauma centre. We then drove the ALS crew back to their ambulance that had been left at the scene. The back of our Ambulance was like a bomb went off: wrappers and opened packages everywhere, littered the floor. We had a big clean-up to do now.

After we dropped 75A1 off at their ambulance, we stopped to chat with the police on scene for a few minutes and found out this was an attempted murder-suicide. The patient we had just airlifted to the trauma centre had attempted to kill his wife. He had shot her twice in the upper body (non-fatally), and then attempted suicide by shooting himself in the head.

I called Dispatch on the cell phone: "We are going to have to go out of service and back to our station to clean up the car, re-stock and download the AED."

Dispatch replied: "Sure no problem, I'll show you out of service and let us know when you are back in service."

"Sure no problem."

On our drive back to the station Sue and I chatted about the call. Sue was incredulous: "I can't believe the that Fire (short term for Fire Department) did not start CPR!"

I replied: "Well, he was shot in the head, found pulseless, and had been down for over ten minutes before they arrived...I don't blame them."

Sue said: "Well it's not obvious death. There is certain criteria for obvious death."

I replied: "Yes, I know, but based on the mechanism of injury (types of events that we use to determine how injured a person is) and his down time, he was dead. I'm surprised we got pulses back. I if it was not for ALS and the drugs we would not have gotten the pulses back. Wonder if he will have brain damage now?"

I never did hear of the outcome of this patient, and whether he survived or not.

MCI

We had just pulled into the station. It was winter and not too cold, but it was the first snow fall in the Lower Mainland, so lots of people were sliding off of roads. I was still sitting in the car when I suddenly heard the hotline (designated direct-line phone to Dispatch with specific ring tone – normally red in color) ring in the station bay. A few moments after, the CAD went "Blip...blip."

I looked at the screen:

- Pre-alert for a MVI
- Unknown injuries, unknown patients
- Respond Code 2

My partner arrived at the car; she was driving today. After she got in, I said: "We have a pre-alert for a MVI at Sidewinder Road and 5th Ave...it's routine for now." She replied: "OK."

As we pulled out, the CAD sounded: "Blip...blip...blip...blip." Every 'blip' signified new information on the display. I read the CAD:

- Head-on collision, two vehicle
- Multiple patients
- FD responding, PD responding

"Great," I said, "head-on collision and we are responding routine... these new dispatch response codes are messed up."

A few moments later the CAD sounded again: "Blip...blip...blip." The CAD read: "Car on fire, 1 person trapped."

I said: "Well they have to upgrade us now...there is a car on fire and one person trapped."

My partner turned the CAD to look at the screen and replied: "Well we can just respond as they gave it to us."

I said: "Well, if they don't upgrade us to Code 3, I'm calling to speak to the D/S[4] about upgrading us.

After a minute with no upgrade, I grabbed the cell phone and called Dispatch.

The dispatcher answered: "Channel 2."

I said: "Yes this is 77 Bravo. We are responding as a single car into a head-on MVI with a car on fire and a trapped person?"

The dispatcher replied: "Yes."

I said: "I want a call review to be done on this, this is crap!"

The dispatcher replied: "Yes I believe there is a number you can call and…" — I interrupted her: "No…now, I want to speak to the D/S." The dispatcher replied: "Oh…OK hold on a minute."

The D/S answered: "Duty Dispatcher Sheri speaking."

"Hi Sheri," I said. "This is 77B responding routine to a head-on MVI, with a car on fire and a trapped person."

Sheri replied: "This should never have been coded like this. Will be upgrading you to Code 3 and see what other resources you will need."

I responded: "OK thanks. Had to call. This is getting a bit crazy with these calls being dispatched like this."

Sheri replied: "Yes just don't take it personally." I said: "Oh, I'm not, just been happening a lot lately. Thanks…talk to you later." I hung up and said: "We are going to be upgraded to Code 3 in a minute."

My partner replied: "We are?"

Just then the CAD sounded — "Blip…blip" — and I read a note to "Respond Code 3 as per the D/S."

I said: "OK we have just been upgraded to Code 3."

My partner turned the CAD and looked at the screen. "Great, Code 3 in these conditions — wet, slippery." She was worried because we know that turning on our emergency equipment can cause accidents because people panic and, when trying to get off the road, can slide into ditches. So, we don't like to turn on the equipment unless absolutely necessary.

I said: "Well, if those people are burned we need to be there."

---

4 Duty Supervisor

My partner activated the emergency equipment and the vehicles ahead of us started to move out of our way as we proceeded to the call. Traffic was moderate and there was a light snow and ice on the roads. As we proceeded to the call the CAD sounded again – "Blip...blip... blip" – and the display read "Helicopter staged, ALS and another BLS unit responding."

It took us approximately 14 minutes to arrive at the call driving Code 3. As we approached, we could see a line of vehicles on the two-lane roadway. I could see a plume of smoke rising in the air when we were ¼ km away. We were waved forward by one of the firefighters on scene, and as we pulled up we could see a full-sized car in the roadway that was smoking and had the entire front-end smashed so badly I could not make out where the engine was. The firefighters were spraying foam on the car. To the right was full-sized pick-up truck in the ditch that had a significant indentation to 50% of the side of the truck. My partner exited and said: "I'll check on the people over there on the other side of the car." I got out and, as I did, a firefighter approached me and began talking.

Firefighter: "OK, I will give you the situation: there is a total of seven patients; a two-year-old – not hurt, was in the car seat; everyone from the car on fire got out OK, so there was four in the car and three in the truck. One guy is trapped in the back and the driver is unconscious out of the truck on the grass."

I was walking to the back to get out equipment as he talked, and replied to him: "We have other units on their way including a helicopter."

I grabbed the kit, the collar bag, and the oxygen, and quickly moved to the side of the truck where the unconscious driver was. A firefighter was beside him. The patient was an East Indian male; he was not moving but had no obvious open wounds or trauma. The firefighter had an oxygen mask on his face.

As I came beside the patient I said to the firefighter: "What do you know about his condition?"

The firefighter replied: "We found him here. He was not responding when I arrived, has a pulse...no obvious injuries."

I moved in to do an assessment and found that the patient responded to pain by moaning. I completed a primary survey with no injuries found. With the help of the firefighter I applied a hard collar, checked his BP, Pulse and Sp02 and blood glucose. His vital signs came back as stable, so I presumed he may have been unbelted and sustained a concussion. In the background I could hear the other patient trapped in the truck, yelling to be let out.

I could hear more sirens in the background and before I knew it there were multiple units on the ground. We had an ALS ambulance, CCT ambulance, two more BLS ambulances, and a supervisor, while a helicopter was en-route.

The driver was packaged, and care was taken over by the CCT Paramedics. I could hear the sound of a helicopter approaching in the distance and was told by the Supervisor that that was our Medi-vac. This patient was loaded into the helicopter and transported to the nearest trauma center.

In the end one patient was Medi-vaced by helicopter, a second patient was transported by ALS, and a third patient was transported by a BLS crew. The profound part of this entire call was that we were dispatched routine with no other resources backing us up. If I had not questioned the MPDS code and spoken to an experienced charge dispatcher we would have arrived to a nightmare beyond our capabilities as a single BLS ambulance.

Don't shoot the messenger

It was a quiet start to the shift. We were sitting at our station relaxing. I had my feet up in our very relaxing easy boy recliners, watching TV and just enjoying the down time. A short time later there was a ringing on the hotline. My partner, who I had worked with often, grabbed the phone.

Todd said: "Are you kidding? Really...a shooting? OK, we will."

I was standing up now with I am sure what was a look of intensity on my face.

Todd looked over smiling now and began to laugh: "You should see the look on your face when I said 'shooting'...ha ha!"

I replied: "Well..."

Todd said: "We have a shooting. It's just up the road a few blocks so we are staged here."

"OK, I replied. "Well, I am going to get some things ready. They will be calling us shortly. I will be out in bay, in the car."

Todd replied: "OK, I'll answer the phone when they call."

"OK, sounds good."

I proceeded out to the bay, went in the back of the Ambulance and set up an IV (1000ml normal saline solution 0.9%), primed the line, and had it ready. I then checked our stock of Asher man chest seals, a special bandage that is used on a chest wound and has a one-way valve that will limit the chances of a tension pneumothorax. We had two in the car and two in the kit, so I thought we were good. I went to the cab of the Amb and looked at the location of the call; it was about 3-4 minutes away.

Just then, the phone rang, and the CAD simultaneously went "Blip...blip...blip...blip," as the new information came across the screen. I reached up and opened the bay door with the remote door opener. Todd arrived shortly afterwards and climbed in. "Looking forward to a shooting, are we?" he said, laughing.

I replied: "Well...could be interesting..."

Todd pulled out, activated the emergency lights, and proceed down the road, turning the siren on as he went. We arrived a few minutes later to a scene of flashing red and blue emergency lights. There must have been eight police cars on scene and one fire truck.

We pulled up and got out. I grabbed the kit and Todd grabbed the O2 and we were directed over to a four-door sedan parked along the roadway. The firefighter began giving me a report.

Firefighter 1: "Looks like a single gunshot wound to the leg."

Me: "OK, is he conscious?"

Firefighter 1: "Yes."

Me: "OK."

I opened the back door of the sedan and saw a young Caucasian male laying on his back partially on his side. Another firefighter was in the back, holding a trauma dressing on his leg.

Me: "Did you check for an exit wound?"

Firefighter 2: "Uh...no."

I asked the firefighter to remove the dressing. The patient still had his jeans on, so I pulled out my scissors and began cutting as I talked to the patient.

"What is your name?"

The patient replied: "Daniel."

I said, "OK, Daniel, what happened?"

Daniel replied: "I was shot in the leg by a guy."

I said: "Were you hit anyplace else? Are you injured anywhere else?

Daniel replied: "No man, just the leg, it fucking hurts man..."

I said: "I bet it does. OK just going to dress this wound then get you out of this car...did you lose consciousness at any time?"

Daniel replied: "No, it all happened so fast!"

I said: "Did you see what type of gun it was?"

Daniel replied: "It was a big fucking handgun man...geez it hurts!"

I cut the man's jeans open and examined his thigh. I could see an entry wound mid-thigh on the front of his leg. The wound was round, approximately 1cm in diameter, with blood oozing from it. I looked and felt behind his leg for an exit wound and could not find one.

I said: "Todd can you grab me a dressing and roller gauze for this wound?"

Todd replied: "Already ahead of you, I have it right here" — Always good when you are working with a partner who is forecasting your thoughts and what you need, especially in a trauma call.

"Perfect, thanks." I grabbed the dressing and wrapped the leg.

When I stepped out of the car, there were people buzzing around everywhere, police cars blocking the area, and bystanders being interviewed. I looked over to my left and noticed a man setting up a video camera on a tripod.

I turned to Todd and said: "Think we need to get this guy out from the other side...the way he is laying we can pull him out." Todd replied: "OK, sounds good. I'll grab the cot and we can pull it up to the door and put him directly onto it."

I said: "Sure, sounds good."

We opened the passenger rear door on the driver's side and adjusted the cot to the height of the car seat. I grabbed beneath Daniel's armpits and pulled him out as Todd and a firefighter stabilized the cot. As I pulled him out, the left leg that had been shot suddenly turned outwards. I realized his femur had been fractured. We strapped him on the cot, applied high-flow O2, and loaded him into the Ambulance. A police officer got in the other side door; as this was a shooting, the police officer was going to accompany us to the hospital. After we got in, Todd came inside and began getting up an IV line as I grabbed the BP cuff and pulse ox. Todd inserted an 18G IV at the AC site and we opened up the flow valve to full wide open to get some fluids in the patient. The potential for shock from blood loss was high as a person can lose a lot of blood if an artery is hit and they can suddenly lose consciousness.

Todd got in and began driving Code 3 to the local trauma hospital, the siren whistling as we went, and bypassing a hospital that was only ten minutes away. We have policy that if specific trauma criteria are met, we will bypass a local hospital and divert to a designated trauma hospital that can properly treat the patient with surgical intervention if required.

I said: "Todd, do we have auto launch on standby for this and ALS?"

He replied: "We have a helo on the pad and ALS is on the way. Do you want to set up a meet?

"Yes, let's set up a meet for ALS. He seems stable but just in case we need them."

Todd replied: "Already taken care of."

"Great!"

After about eight minutes Todd told me that we were getting close to the ALS meeting point. He stopped the car and within moments two ALS paramedics entered the back. I knew the attendant well. The ALS paramedic (Don) said: "Hey Luc what have you got?" I explained the story to him: that it was a single GSW to his left leg, the leg was broken, and vitals were stable.

Don said: "OK let's go. I don't think there is anything I need to do for him but will come along for the ride if anything changes. I will need one of you to drive our car in for us, do you mind?"

I responded: "OK, sounds good, no not at all."

Todd handed me his keys, and they drove away sirens blazing.

The ride to the trauma hospital was uneventful and the patient remained stable en route. I followed routine and arrived at the trauma hospital ten minutes after they did. It was later discovered from the x-ray that the bullet hit the patient's femur and shattered it. In fact, the bullet fragments could be seen inside his leg.

After we cleaned up our car and re-stocked, we re-entered the front cab area of the ambulance.

"Well, that was fun!" said Todd.

I replied: "Yes, it was. Have not done a shooting in a while."

92-year-old Hug

It was still early, and we received a routine call to the hospital, asking us to transfer a patient home. We arrived at the local hospital and checked in with the ER PCC.[5] She advised us that the patient was in bed #3 and was ready to go home. I was attending this evening and received a report from the bedside nurse. The patient was a 92-year-old woman who had suffered a fall, two days previously. She had received minor skin tears on her arms, but x-rays proved that there were no fractures. She had been kept in hospital due to a UTI (urinary tract infection) and had received IV antibiotics.

I went to the bedside and greeted the patient.

"Hi Mrs. Brown, how are you feeling?

---

5   Patient Care Coordinator

The patient replied: "I want to get home now."

I said: "Well we can certainly do that. What is the best way to get you onto our stretcher?"

She replied: "Well, I can stand."

"Do you normally use a walker?" I asked.

Mrs. Brown replied: "Well dear, yes I do but get along OK on my own."

I said: "I'm sure you do, but we will help you get on the cot. My partner and I will just use a blanket lift to move you over. Just give yourself a hug and we will take care of the rest OK?"

The patient replied: "Oh I don't want to be a bother."

I said: "No bother, it's full service today. Just relax we will take care of everything."

My partner and I used a blanket lift to move the 100lb woman onto our cot. We loaded her up and took the short eight-minute drive to the patient's independent living residential building. When we assisted her off our cot onto the carpet she turned to me. "I want to give my handsome paramedic a hug. Thank you so much for all of your help" She gave me a big hug – and I returned it.

I think if the lighting was a bit brighter there might have been a slight blush on my face.

I replied: "You are so welcome. Anytime we can help."

We waited until the patient was inside her residence and said a final goodbye.

As we left, I said to my partner: "I don't mind doing transfers home like that. That lady was so appreciative, and she certainly can't get home on her own."

My partner replied: "Yeah, no kidding. Wish all our transfers home were like that."

Pedestrian Struck – Thrown into Ditch

I was working at a station in the Fraser Valley. We were at our station when suddenly the pagers sounded: "Beep...Beep...Beep...shhhhhh-hh...08Alpha2... Code 3 call...08A2 Code 3...shhhhhhh."

Went went out to the car and my partner, who was driving, called in: "08A2 – we are 10-8."

Dispatch responded: "08A2 Code 3 MVA. Head on collision at Perimeter Road and Cross. Two cars, multiple patients, unknown injuries at this time. Fire and police responding...we are looking at getting you ALS from quarters, but they are thirty minutes out."

My partner (Bob) replied: "10-4."

We pulled out of the bay and Bob activated all the emergency equipment. We drove away from the station with the siren wailing.

It was a dark, early evening on a summer day, and it was cool but not cold.

The radio squawked: "08A2."

Bob replied: "08A2."

Dispatch: "08A2 – 5s on scene say that there are at least four patients including a pedestrian struck. We are launching 90V (helicopter) and getting you another couple BLS cars."

My partner replied: "10-4."

As we pulled up to the scene, I could see that we were the first emergency vehicle on scene, although it took us eight minutes to respond. I could hear the sirens of the Fire Department in the distance. As we surveyed the scene, we could see two cars that had been in a collision and people milling about them. In the distance down a grass median we could see a few other people milling about. A man walked up frantically and said: "There is a guy who is hurt down there" — he pointed to a few people in the grass median — "I think he was hit by one of these cars."

My partner said: "I'm going to check out the people in the cars, if you want to check out who is hurt in the median."

I grabbed the kit and headed to the median with a hard collar in hand. When I arrived, I found a man who was laying on the grass with part of his left leg still sitting in a puddle of standing water. There was a firefighter with him. The patient was conscious and complaining of pain on the right side of his chest and leg. He was breathing at a rate of approximately 28 breaths-per-minute. I found out that he had been hit by a car and thrown over thirty feet into the median! I could not believe he was conscious. I was alone with the firefighter and a bystander. As I looked up at the roadway, another ambulance was pulling up and I could see the words "Advanced Life Support Paramedic" on the side. I did not know how many patients there were in total.

I directed my questions to the patient: "Did you lose consciousness?"

He replied: "I don't think so. My leg is killing me, can you give me something for pain?"

I replied: "I can't give you anything right now, but when I get you into the Ambulance I will give you something for the pain, First I want to move you out of this water. With the help of the firefighter we slid him back, pulling his lower leg from the water.

I continued with my trauma assessment, systematically going from head to toe by assessing his chest, auscultating breath sounds, palpating his body, and checking for open wounds. To my surprise, his injuries were only to his left side where the car struck him, and he didn't appear to have any serious life-threatening injuries. I told the firefighter I was going back to the Ambulance for the clam and some blankets. When I returned I packaged the patient, splinting his leg with blankets between his legs and Velcro trauma straps. I wanted to do simple stabilization and get him inside the Ambulance where I could assess him properly in the warm, lit patient compartment. With the help of a couple other firefighters, we carried the man on the clam to the cot I had pulled out of the Ambulance.

We loaded him in the back and I began a secondary assessment, cutting his jeans off to access his leg better. He continued to be in severe pain ("10 out of 10"), and I began prepping to start an IV as I heard the sound of rotor blades. They had called in a helicopter for a medi-vac; there must have been someone who was in serious trouble. I was still alone in the back of the Ambulance and wondered where my partner was. I opened the back doors and called out for some help. A firefighter arrived, and I told him I needed an ALS for pain management. I continued my secondary trauma assessment looking closer for any injuries I had not found. I grabbed the BP cuff and was just about to take the patient's blood pressure when the back doors opened again and now two firefighters were standing there.

"Where is the ALS paramedic?" I asked them.

One of the firefighters replied: "He said he was busy with a sick patient."

I said: "Really? So rather than come by and find out why I need him he just ignores me? Can you go back and tell him I need pain management for this guy now!?"

While they went away, I finished getting the patient's vitals (blood pressure, pulse and respirations). I waited another five minutes and still nobody showed up. I turned to the firefighter who was in the back with me and said, "I am going to get someone." He nodded as I exited the back of the Ambulance. I looked around: to my left there was a helicopter on the ground, and to my right I could see three other ambulances. There was what appeared to be four paramedics working on a lady sitting in the front passenger seat of a car. I thought to myself 'It is taking four paramedics to treat one patient and I am in the back of the Ambulance with a guy who was struck by a car and thrown at least thirty feet into the median?'

I walked over to my partner and said: "Hey, I need some help in the back of the car. Need pain management. He was hit by a car and thrown thirty feet."

My partner replied: "We have a very sick patient in that car, might be a bit."

I said: "How many ALS does it take? You have CCT and ALS all working on one patient?" I shook my head. "Just send someone over, and we have to roll soon." Bob — looking rather dumbfounded — replied: "OK."

I walked back to the car, quickly entered the back of the Ambulance, and re-checked the patient's condition. Although I only had six years of experience as a paramedic at this time, with all my experience as a medic and trauma first aid instructor I knew that with mechanism of injury alone this guy could have internal injuries and crash at any time. I wanted him in a hospital if he did.

Suddenly, the back doors of the Ambulance opened, and there was an ALS paramedic standing there. "I heard you called for me."

I replied: "Yeah, I did, a couple times. This guy is in severe pain, was thrown thirty feet into that median, and needs pain management."

He climbed in: "You don't even have an IV going yet," he said, looking at me with a frown. "We have been dealing with a very sick patient."

I replied: "Yeah, I heard, and I have been in the back of this car by myself doing an assessment on a guy hit by a car, and you have two CCT and two ALS on one patient."

The ALS paramedic was clearly pissed off at me, but I didn't care at this point. He started an IV and asked the patient a few questions. He then turned to me and said: "He can wait on pain management until you get to the hospital."

I looked at him in disbelief and said: "You have got to be kidding me?"

The ALS paramedic said, "Nope," and exited the back of the Ambulance.

The firefighter looked at me and said: "Nice guy."

I replied: "Yeah, a real charmer he is."

The doors opened in the back of the Ambulance; it was my partner Bob standing there. "Are you ready to go?" he asked.

"Yes," I said, "we need to get going now."

Bob replied, "OK," closed the back doors of the Ambulance, and entered the cab up front. The firefighter asked: "Do you still need me?

I said: "No, thanks, I should be good. The hospital is only eight minutes away, and he is stable at the moment."

The firefighter exited through the back doors and we began to move. Bob called back to me from the front and said: "Are you OK with routine?" I replied: "Yes, routine is fine for now. I will let you know."

"Sounds good."

The patient remained in extreme pain — "10 out of 10," as he put it — on the way to the hospital. I offered him Entonox en route, but it did little for his pain. After arriving at the hospital, we off loaded the patient in the trauma room.

I was certainly a bit disappointed by how this call played out. My patient could have been in serious condition and none of the other paramedics on scene even came to check how I was doing during the assessment, extrication and secondary in the back of the Ambulance. Bob and I didn't talk about the call and just continued back to the station until our next call came in.

Hide and Seek

It was early afternoon and my partner (Jeff) and I were working in a rural station on call-out. (This meant we only got paid when we got paged out on our voice pagers). We were chillin'; Jeff was reading, and I was making some lunch when suddenly the pagers screeched: "Beep beep beep beep beep....shhhhhhh....88Kilo Code 3 call...88Kilo Code 3."

Jeff was closer to the phone, so he walked over and called Dispatch.

He got off the phone and said: "We have a Code 3 call for a short-of-breath five-year-old, possibly trapped."

I replied: "Trapped?" with a confused expression on my face. "Did he say where the child was trapped, and do we have Fire?"

Jeff replied: "He did not say either."

"OK," I said. "Guess we better get dressed then get going on this."

We both quickly changed into our uniforms and headed out to the Ambulance parked in the bay. Jeff was driving, and I acknowledged and pushed the 'En Route' button our call on an older style of CAD system.

After leaving the bay, Jeff activated the emergency lights and, after turning down the only road through town, he activated the siren: "Yeeeeeooooow...yeeeeeeeoooow." I hate sirens. Even though the ambulances are soundproofed, I always carry a pair of ear protection especially for long stat (emergency) transfers.

Jeff accelerated, and I could hear the engine strain as we accelerated above the posted speed limit. Traffic was light as we entered the main highway. The call was approximately 18 kilometres away. When we arrived, we could see a small ranch-style house. There was a abandoned car, a washing machine, and another unidentifiable appliance on the lawn. (This house was on First Nations reserve land and these sights were typical in this area).

We were greeted at the door by an eight-year-old Native girl. She directed us to where her friend was. We entered a small laundry room with a top loading washer and dryer. To my surprise there was a girl inside the top loading washer. As I approached, I could see the panic in her eyes. I took a look at her skin color: it was pink, she did not appear in respiratory distress, and there were no obvious wounds or bleeding.

I said "Hi, what is your name?"

She replied: "Ashley."

"How old are you?"

"Seven."

"Why did you climb in there?" I asked.

Ashley replied: "We were playing hide and seek, and I climbed in here then got stuck."

"I see. Well we are going to have to get you out of there."

I grasped her under her shoulders and attempted to pull her out. The center post of the washer was pressing against her chest and she was jammed in.

My partner had already gotten out the pulse ox (pulse and oxygen saturation monitor). I placed it on her finger...it displayed a pulse of 122 with a O2 sat of 98%.

I said: "Are you having any trouble breathing, or are you in any pain?"

Ashley replied: "Well this thing" (she pointed to the centre post on the washer) "is pushing against my chest and it hurts a bit."

I said: "Don't worry we are going to get you out OK."

Ashley nodded.

I said to the other girl: "Are there any tools in the house?"

She replied: "I don't know."

I looked at my partner and said "Looks like we are going to have to dis-assemble this washer to get her out. Can you get Fire started just in case we cannot find any way of removing this top?"

My partner replied: "Sure sounds good, what are you thinking?"

I had looked around the rim of the washer and noticed some screws that were holding the top down.

I replied: "Looks like if we can remove these four screws, we can remove the top and we should be able to get her out."

Jeff grabbed his radio and made a call: "22 Kilo."

Dispatch: "22 Kilo."

Jeff replied: "22 Kilo can you start Fire? We have a seven-year-old girl trapped in a washing machine and may need some assistance to get her out."

Dispatch: "Do you require them Code 3?"

My partner replied: "10-4."

I turned to my partner and said "I have a Leatherman tool in my bag in the car. I will go get it. It has a small Phillips screwdriver on it that might work." He replied: "OK."

I returned with my Leatherman and luckily it had a Phillips screwdriver that fit. I began to unscrew the lid.

Ashley said: "My chest is starting to hurt more now...I want to get out."

"We will get you out very soon," I replied.

My partner turned on the O2 and placed a mask on the girl without me saying anything.

I remarked: "Great idea, she is sating good, but won't hurt to get some more O2 in her until we can get her out."

It took me fifteen minutes to unscrew all the screws as the Leatherman tool was not the best for the job, but worked in the end. Once all of the screws were removed, we were able to remove the outer lid and top of the washer and that gave us enough space between the centre post and washer tub to pull her out.

The Fire Department arrived just as we pulled her out. The girl's mother also showed up, as she had been at a neighbour's while the kids played. After a check-up and check for injuries, I advised the mother that we should take her to the hospital for a more thorough check-up. The mother agreed. We transported Ashley and her mother to the local hospital without further incident.

As we departed the hospital I said: "Well that is a first for me."

Jeff replied: "No kidding — never seen that happen before."

Sixteen-year-old Anaphylaxis

We were almost off shift, sitting at our station hoping that the we would have a break from our busy day in Surrey. The phone hotline suddenly rang. We were 'up car' so I answered the red phone on the wall.

"Hey, it's a pre-alert," I said to my partner.

My partner responded: "Ah figures — just when we get a minute of downtime we get a call. Well let's get it done."

I said: "Yeah, well maybe it will be a good call for Joanne."

My student (Joanne) was only in her first week of on-car practicum but was doing very well and picking up on the skills very early on. She would make a good Paramedic.

Hearing her name, Joanne said: "Yes, I hope so."

We all headed out to the bay. I was attending and my partner driving. After getting inside I spun the CAD and looked at the screen.

It read:

- Code 3
- 16 yo Female anaphylaxis

- previous history of nut allergy
- facial swelling developing, throat swelling
- FD responding

I pushed the 'En Route' button and spun the CAD to my partner and he read the information. "Looks like the real deal, on this one," he said. "Yeah, no kidding!"

My partner pulled out of the bay turned on the emergency lights and siren as we pulled onto the roadway. The residence was only a short six-minute drive away.

The radio crackled: "76A2 no ALS available, just you and the Fire." My partner replied: "10-4."

The student, Joanne, was peering through the open area from the back seat as my partner drove quickly to the call. This could be a true life-threatening emergency, so seconds would count. We pulled up to a residence a few minutes later and my partner said: "You head up. I will grab the O2."

"Sounds good," I replied, and exited the Ambulance with Joanne behind me with the jump kit.

We arrived at the door and were greeted by a black man. He said: "It's my daughter. We think she ate something with nuts in it and she is very allergic to them."

I said: "OK, lead the way."

We followed him upstairs to a bedroom. When we entered there was a young black girl sitting on the bed, but she was in no obvious distress. A black woman (who later we would find out was her mother) was next to her.

As we walked into the room I let Joanne begin questioning the girl. "Hi, my name is Joanne, what is your name?"

The girl replied; "Megan"

Joanne said: "Hi Megan, are you having any difficulty breathing right now?"

Megan replied: "I am feeling tightness in my throat, and it's starting to feel a bit restrictive."

I had opened the jump bag at this point and had the SPO2 monitor in my hand as well as the BP cuff.

When Joanne looked back at me I handed them to her and said: "Grab a quick pressure."

She replied: "OK."

Joanne placed the SPO2 monitor on Megan's finger and I noticed the bright red LED display numbers: Pulse:135 O2 stats 98%. I made a mental note of the numbers as I began to pull out the medication box.

Joanne finished the BP and said: "Her blood pressure is 110/68."

I replied: "OK, her vitals are stable at this point. Is there anything else you want to do or ask her?"

Joanne replied: "Yes." At this point the mother said: "She ate some cake at a party and we think there may have been nuts in it."

I said: "How long has it been since she ate the cake?"

The mother replied: "Thirty-five minutes ago."

"Has she vomited at all?" I asked.

The mother replied; "Yes, after she vomited then she started feeling tightness in her throat."

"Megan," I asked, "has the tightness gotten worst since this happened?"

Megan nodded as she said: "Yes, it's feeling very tight."

Looking at the mother, I asked: "Did you give her an EpiPen?"

The mother replied: "No, the one we had just expired. We also wanted to see how she was before giving it to her. After she vomited and started feeling her throat tighten we called 911."

My partner was completing paperwork during our questioning.

I said: "Sorry Joanne, continue with our assessment and questions."

I turned back to the medication box, removed a 1cc ampule of epinephrine, a 1cc syringe and alcohol swab. I knew we had to administer Epi immediately based on this girl's history.

Joanne continued asking a few more pertinent questions relating to the girl's history.

I said: "Joanne did you auscultate her lungs"

She replied: "No, not yet."

I said: "Maybe do that now. Find out if there is any restriction in her lungs."

I handed my partner the oral Benadryl to measure up. When Joanne finished auscultating, she turned back to me; I was holding the 1cc syringe of Epi and an alcohol swab. She looked at me in surprise.

"So how do her lungs sound?" I asked.

Joanne replied: "They sound OK — a bit of expiratory wheezing in the upper lobes."

I said: "OK, here is 0.3mg Epi. Inject her with this."

Joanne looked a bit shocked again and said: "I don't feel comfortable with that."

I said: "You practiced in class did you not?"

Joanne responded: "We practiced on oranges."

In the background I could hear other sirens getting closer. I assumed it was the Fire Department as the ALS unit was not available. To Joanne I said: "It will be OK, just swab her arm, inject it in like a dart, and administer the Epi."

Joanne replied: "Can you, do it?"

I said: "Sure, she needs it now so let me get in closer and give it to her." I injected the patient with the Epi and said: "OK, we should get going to the hospital. Do you think you can walk down the stairs?"

Megan nodded and said: "Yes, I am sure I can."

I heard some noise downstairs; it was the Fire Department. I called out: "Hey guys we are coming down, can you grab the cot from the car and set it up please? We have to roll on this one."

I heard a male voice: "Sure we will take care of it."

My partner, who had measured the oral Benadryl, was standing there holding it.

I said to Megan: "My partner is going to give you some oral Benadryl to help offset the allergic reaction."

Megan replied: "OK."

My partner handed Megan the small medicine cup with a dose of Benadryl. After Megan took it I said: "OK, ready to go?"

We began helping the girl down the stairs. By the time we got to the bottom of the stairs, the cot had been set up by the firefighters. There were three of them; two were wearing turnout pants. Megan was helped on the cot, buckled in, and loaded into the Ambulance. I took a moment to auscultate her chest to verify what Joanne had heard and Megan definitely had expiratory wheezing to the upper lobes of her lungs.

We departed for the closest hospital. As we did, my partner said: "Routine or Code 3?"

I replied: "Code 3, and can you hand me the cell please?"

My partner handed me the cell phone through the opening from the front cab to the rear patient compartment area. Megan's mother was sitting in the front of the Ambulance with my partner.

"Is ALS available if we need them?" I asked my partner.

My partner contacted Dispatch and we were told that ALS was still not available. We then headed to the hospital, which was approximately ten to fourteen minutes away.

Turning to Joanne, I asked: "OK, is there anything else we need to do?"

Joanne replied: "Well, we can continue to monitor her, take another BP?"

I said: "Great idea, you get a pressure and I will notify the hospital."

I flipped the older style flip-phone open, found the number to the ER triage at the hospital we were heading to, and hit send.

After a few rings a woman answered the phone: "Triage."

I said: "Hi this is Luciano with BC Ambulance. We are heading in Code 3 with a sixteen-year-old female patient with a severe nut allergy. It is believed she consumed some nuts about 43 minutes ago and has since been experiencing increased tightness in the throat and chest with expiratory wheezing. Her vitals are stable this time. We have initiated treatment of 0.3mg Epi IM and 50mg oral Benadryl. Our ETA is about ten minutes."

The triage nurse said: "OK thanks we will be ready when you get here"

I replied: "Great, thanks, see you soon."

Joanne had finished taking the patient's blood pressure at this point. She looked over at me and said: "Her BP is 105/50."

I turned to Megan and said: "How are you feeling? How is your throat feeling?"

Megan replied: "It feels like it is still getting tighter and more restrictive."

I auscultated her lungs again and could still hear the expiratory wheezing.

I picked up the phone and called our physician on call for repeat Epi orders. With our current treatment guidelines, we were only permitted to give one dose of Epi. We were required to call our physician on call for order of more medication.

I discussed the situation with the doctor and told him that I wanted to give a second dose of 0.3mg Epi. He agreed.

I turned to Joanne and said: "Can you draw up 0.3mg Epi please?"

Joanne looked surprised and replied: "Um, I would feel better if you did it."

I said: "OK, but this is the best opportunity to get some practice in, when you have a preceptor in the Ambulance with you."

I grabbed a new ampule, snapped off the glass end, inserted a one-inch needle attached to a 1cc syringe, and drew up 0.3cc (0.3mg) of epinephrine. I said to Joanne: "OK, do you want to give this dose?"

Joanne looked at me with a sort of fear in her eyes and replied: "No, I would rather you just did it." I was a bit disappointed at this point as I wanted Joanne to get the experience of giving an injection under the supervision of a preceptor, rather than experience the first time on her own after she was licensed.

I exposed Megan's arm, swabbed the skin, and inserted the needle into her arm like a dart. After administering the second dose, we continued to the hospital Code 3. On the way, the girl began showing signs of improvement. I was surprised how calm she was.

After we arrived at the hospital, we were triaged and gave hand-over to the bedside nurse. We then headed back to the car to clean up, make up the cot and discuss the call. On the way back, I said to Joanne: "So, what did you think of that?"

Joanne replied: "I was a bit overwhelmed by everything. It all went so fast. I was trying to think of all my treatment guidelines and what to do."

I said: "Well, you don't see full blown anaphylaxis very often. We get a fair amount of allergic reactions, but few anaphylaxes. So, to be able to see that during your precepting is pretty good experience and exposure."

My partner who was with us pushing the cot said: "Yeah, no kidding. We certainly don't see very many anaphylaxis. You got a good call."

I turned to Joanne again and said: "So, why didn't you want to give the Epi injection?"

Joanne replied: "Well I was...just didn't feel comfortable with it. We practiced with oranges in the class, and now this was a real person, who was in crisis. I just felt overwhelmed with everything. Seemed like everything was going so fast."

I said: "Well, at least you were able to experience it. Many paramedics work years without actually seeing a true anaphylaxis patient."

Junior mints

While working in a busy urban area early one evening, we were on our way to a routine call when the radio squawked: "98A2."

My partner replied: "98A2."

"98A2 cancel previous and take instead."

I grabbed the pen and pad and got ready to write. The dispatcher read out the call: "19345 Dawson Street, the Complex movie theatre. It's Code 3 for an unconscious male, cardiac arrest. CPR in progress; staff will meet you at the entrance. You are with 96A1 from quarters. Fire is responding."

My partner activated the emergency lights and turned on the siren. "I have not done an arrest in a while," my partner commented.

I replied: "Yeah, me neither. Weird how calls like this come in waves; you get a few in a row then nothing for a while."

Traffic was moderately heavy as my partner zipped around cars, changing the siren tones often as he drove. We arrived outside the theatre a few minutes later. There was a fire truck parked outside with all its emergency lights flashing. The second advanced life support ambulance (96A1) had not arrived yet. We got out, and I went for the kit as my partner began to unload the cot. We loaded on the kit, O2, AED, portable suction, and hung the clamshell on the side of the cot and proceeded to the entrance. A staff member was waiting for us as we approached.

I asked: "Do you know what happened?"

The staff member replied: "No, just that a guy watching the movie collapsed. My manager is upstairs and knows more."

My partner replied: "OK thanks."

We were guided into an elevator and along a corridor to the movie theatre entrance. There were a few people milling about that had come out of the theatres. We entered the theatre, and the lights had been turned up, but it was still dim. The firefighters were performing chest compressions on a rather large Caucasian man, whose chest was bare. Their AED was connected to his chest. There was one firefighter at his head with a BVM.

As we approached, the Captain spoke: "Hi guys, this is a thirty-seven-year-old man, who apparently collapsed in his seat during the movie. It took a while for anyone to realize it."

The manager, who was also standing nearby, said: "Apparently from other people in the theatre the man was coughing, then stopped. It was not until the staff came in to clean up the garbage that they found he was collapsed in his chair and not breathing. It was at least fifteen minutes, maybe longer."

As we moved down to assess the patient's airway and pulses I asked: "So do we know how long he was unconscious?" My partner began to get an OPA out and get our suction ready. The manager replied to my query: "No, not really...could have been over ten minutes."

I turned to my partner: "Can you hand me a red airway and the suction, there is foam coming from this guy's mouth."

He replied, "Sure," and handed me the suction and airway.

I began to suction the patient's mouth that was all filled with a white foam. Just then, the ALS (Advanced Life Support) crew arrived. I recognized them as they approached.

One of the the ALS guys (Bob) said: "Hey guys what cycle are you on right now?"

The Fire Captain replied: "Just starting the third."

My partner added: "And no shocks."

The other ALS paramedic (Joe) began to connect their monitor to the patient.

Bob said: "How's that airway Luciano?"

I replied: "It sucks, this guy has this white foam in his mouth, and I can't get any good air movement when I vent him, think you will need to check this out."

Bob replied: "OK, I'll grab my intubation kit."

I caught Bob up on the situation. "Apparently the staff found him after the movie ended. He had been coughing during the movie then stopped at some point. No one really knows how long down he was unresponsive. Sounds like it was over fifteen minutes."

Bob replied sarcastically: "Great."

We continued working on the man in the isle of the theatre. Here was a guy who was at a movie by himself. He was enjoying some junior mints and one or more lodged in his airway. I am sure he began hacking or making unusual movements that others around him would have noticed but they had no idea this man was choking to death. Once this man stopped moving, nobody in the theatre thought anything different, as they were focused on the movie. When the movie was over, and people saw him sitting there, not moving, did they think he was asleep? Perhaps there were only a few people in the theatre that evening, and people exited quickly, not paying attention. Whatever happened, nobody knew until staff came around after the movie to clean up to find that this man was unconscious, not breathing, and in cardiac arrest.

We continued to work the call past the thirty-minute mark. This is normally the determining point that if we do not get a return of spontaneous pulses we call a physician and request instructions to stop resuscitation efforts. Even though here had been a delay in finding the man, we did not have an exact time of cardiac arrest. Due to his young age and viable heart we continued to almost an hour.

Bob finally said: "OK, guys we have been here almost an hour. We have tried everything. Does anyone have any idea of anything we have not done before I call the physician?"

We all looked around at each other and nobody said anything. Bob stepped away and made a call; he spoke for a few minutes, then came back.

Bob said: "OK, you can stop CPR."

The firefighter at the chest just stopped compressing, the person at the airway stopped bagging the patient. There is always a moment of pause after we stop resuscitation efforts. Everyone is probably simply just taking in everything we did. We had just worked on this guy for almost an hour trying to save him and we were not successful. We all knew this was out of our control, but we are rescuers — that is what we do that is why we picked our careers; it was not for the money.

We began cleaning all our equipment up, tying off IV lines so they would not leak. Defibulator pads, intubation tubes and IVs had to be left in place for the coroner as part of their post mortem investigation.

As we rolled our cot back with all our equipment I thought about this call. This guy died in a theatre surrounded by other people and died as nobody knew he was choking to death. It seemed almost unbelievable.

We called Dispatch and put our car out of service until we could clean up the equipment (suction etc.).

This call left an impact on me for a long time afterwards; not because of his death, but because he died surrounded by other people who, if they knew, could have saved his life.

Roll-over Ejection

It was the start of the shift. We had just done our morning checks on the car and the pagers sounded "…Beep beep beep beep…shhhhhhhhh…93A Code 3 call, Code 3 call." My partner picked up the hotline and a few moments later hung up.

He said: "We have a Code 3 for a rollover MVA."

I was driving this morning. We got in and rolled out of the station. I called Dispatch on the radio: "93A we are 10-8."

Dispatch: "10-4…I am starting 92A1 from quarters and we are staging a helicopter. Sounds like it's an ejection."

I replied: "10-4."

I activated the (lights and siren) and proceed to the call. Traffic was still light, it was a clear day, and the roads were very frosty from the morning dew.

The call was on a rural road approximately ten to twelve minutes from the station.

Although I was careful with driving in the frosty road, I pushed it a bit to get us there. This call sounded serious, but we had to make sure we got there safely; if we got into an accident responding to this call, we would be no good to anyone injured and a car farther away would have to respond to this call (and possibly us). Driving Code 3 did give me a small adrenaline rush but not like when I first started; now it was about getting there as fast and as safe as possible. Often, when traffic is heavy, and people do not move out of our way or do things like block us, it becomes more of a frustration.

As we proceed to the call I thought about what we would do on scene if it was in fact a roll-over ejection. More often than not when calls come in they are reported as something and when we arrive on scene it is completely different.

My partner and I didn't chat much on the way to this call.

As I made a turn from a main two-lane roadway onto a rural road I could feel the Ambulance slip slightly, as it was very slippery on the roads that morning. I could see the frost covering the undriven road as we proceeded to the call.

As we approached, we could see a vehicle pulled to the side of the road to the left and to the right another vehicle was on its side against a fence. There was debris scattered around the vehicle. As we pulled up, I noticed a man lying beside the roadway. He was not moving, and I could see visible blood around his head and face. Another man was kneeling beside him. I pulled up just past the rolled over truck and stopped.

I grabbed the radio: "93A 10-7. Single vehicle roll-over. Will advise."

Dispatch: "10-4, 94A1 is six minutes out. A helicopter is staged. Advise if they are required to launch."

I replied: "10-4."

We moved toward the man on the ground and the man kneeling beside him began talking: "I came across this truck, and it looks like this guy was ejected out of the truck. He is breathing but I cannot wake him up."

My partner moved in to access the patient. He called out: "Grab the suction and the spinal kit."

I retrieved the equipment and when I returned he was measuring an OPA (Oral pharyngeal airway). He inserted the airway, and we placed the patient on high flow O2 15lpm via non-rebreather mask. I began to get a blood pressure, and we connected the O2 Sat monitor... it displayed a sat of 98%. Good — he was sating adequately. His blood pressure was 90/40, which was low, but still adequate. We could hear the sirens in the distance.

Using my portable radio, I called Dispatch: "93A."

Dispatch: "93A."

I replied: "93A we require the helicopter. There is a field adjacent to where we are."

Dispatch: "10-4."

Just then, the Fire Department pulled up. The crew came over I spoke to the Captain: "Cap, we are going to need an LZ (landing zone) set up in that field, we have a chopper inbound."

The Fire Captain replied: "OK no problem. Is there anything else we can do to help?"

I said: "We are going to get this guy in our car asap. He is very cold. ALS will be here shortly. We may need some help packaging him."

The Captain replied: "OK I will get a couple of my guys to help you and the other will begin setting up the LZ."

I said: "Great, thanks."

I could hear sirens again in the background and looked up to see another ambulance approaching in the distance.

I went back over to where my partner was with the patient. He had placed a hard collar on the man and had the clam lying beside him. The firefighters came over to help as we assembled the equipment. I had grabbed a blanket from the car and placed it over the patient to help keep him warm.

Just then, the ALS car pulled up and the crew got out and came over to us. The attending ALS paramedic said: "How many patients are there? Is this the only one?"

My partner replied: "Yes, just him."

ALS paramedic: "We need to get this guy in the back of your car. He is very cold."

We all packaged the patient onto the clam and placed him on the stretcher and inside the back of the heated car. The heaters had been placed on high to pre-heat the compartment. After the patient was loaded we trauma-stripped the man and placed blankets over him. We began looking for veins to start an IV as the ALS paramedics began prepping his intubation kit.

I heard the radio squawk: "77V...we are 10min ETA, is there an LZ set up?"

I heard the Fire Captain reply: "77V...Fire...we have an LZ set up in the field adjacent to the scene of the accident."

The ALS paramedic said: "We are going to have to get ready to move up to meet the air evac crew. Who is driving?"

I replied: "I am. I'll leave you guys with this and get ready. Just let me know when you are ready to move."

After exiting the back of the car, I walked over to take a closer look at the pickup truck the patient had been in. It clearly rolled at least once before coming to rest on its side. It was clear to me that the patient had not been wearing his seat belt at the time of the accident.

I got back in the driver's seat and waited for the word. The police had arrived while we had been in the back working on the patient and blocked off the area. A few minutes later the ALS paramedic said: "OK, we are good to move to the road adjacent to the LZ."

After stopping the car, I got out. I could hear the 'clack clack clack' of the helicopter's blades as it approached the LZ. The helicopter circled the LZ then set up his approach. After the helicopter landed and the rotors stopped turning, the air-evac crew walked over with their equipment. They went in the back and began hand-over with the ALS crew and initiated their own treatment.

Now we waited. I stayed outside of the back of our car as there were four paramedics in the back, one ALS, and two air flight paramedics.

Time began to tick. As we passed an hour on scene, I began to wonder what was taking so long with getting this guy ready for flight. I asked the ALS paramedic when he exited the back. He told me they were having trouble intubating the patient. I thought about this, as we had O2 sats of 98% when we arrived on scene.

Finally, the back of the Ambulance doors opened. I looked inside to see the man intubated with an IV running, wrapped in a pressure infuser. We unloaded the patient and with six of us moved the stretcher to the helicopter sitting idle in the field.

We loaded the patient, ventilating him with a BVM as he was loaded into the helicopter. We moved back and got back into our ambulance and moved to a place we could see the helicopter take off. We always stay until it departs just in case something happens on lift-off and they have to do an emergency landing, or, even worse, crash on lift-off.

After the helicopter took off I heard the pilot say: "77V ETA to trauma centre fifteen minutes."

I looked at my watch and calculated the time since our arrival: 1 hour, 47 minutes. If you added the time the accident happened and our travel time to the scene it was easily over two hours since the crash. What made this worse is that we could have travelled by road to the trauma centre in 45 minutes or less from where we were.

I said to my partner: "So much for the golden hour! I can't believe they stayed on the ground for almost two hours just to intubate him."

He replied: "Well they have a policy that they have to intubate prior to flying as they can't intubate in the air."

I said: "Yeah...and last week I transported a guy by myself in the back, with an active bleed from his mouth in the lateral C-spine position so he would not aspirate...and did that on a rough logging road...it's BS that they have to intubate prior to flying!!"

My partner replied: "Well, maybe so but that's how they do it."

We departed the scene and didn't say much on our way back to the station, both of us processing the events of the call.

A week later as I read the paper, I noticed a small article that explained how a man who was ejected from a roll-over MVA died of his injuries. I knew this was the same accident as they listed the road of the accident. I will never know if the delay in transport to a trauma centre was the cause of death.

Following too close

We were relaxing in the station when the hotline rang. My partner answered the phone, turned to me, and said: "We have an MVI Hwy #23 routine."

I replied: "Yeah, ever since they changed the response codes, all MVI are 'routine.' Well we can just take our time and head out there. If there is anything serious they can upgrade us."

My partner replied: "Oh...sure we'll take our time."

Today was my drive day, so I jumped into the driver's seat, my partner operated the CAD, and we headed out. We were approximately fifteen minutes from the call, routine. As my partner looked at the CAD, he told me what it read: "It says three-car MVI...police on scene...unknown injuries at this time."

As I entered the busy highway with morning commuters the traffic backed up quickly and we began moving at a crawl of only 15km/h. "I'm going to light it up to get through this traffic or we will never make it," I said.

My partner replied: "Sure, sounds good to me."

I activated the emergency equipment and, with the siren wailing, drove down the centre of the two-lane highway, splitting the traffic. Vehicles began to respond and moved to the left and right of me, opening a path down the middle of the lanes. We were still moving slowly — approximately 30-50km/h, as the traffic was almost chalked to a dead stop.

The CAD sounded again — "Blip...blip" — and my partner looked at the screen and said: "It says all persons walking on scene. Looks like this is going to be a minor MVI. Probably just check everyone out." I nodded in agreement. As I continued driving, I noticed headlights in my mirrors closing in to our rear. A vehicle was shadowing us as we went through traffic.

"Look at this jerk shadowing us," I said. "Guess he thinks he does not have to wait like everyone else this morning. What an ass. I should stop."

My partner looked in his mirror and then looked over at me: "Yes you should."

That was all I needed: my partner to agree with me. I stopped the Ambulance, and my partner looked over at me with a slight look of disbelief. I got out, with all the traffic stopped and the emergency lights flashing. I walked directly toward a full-sized pickup truck stopped a short distance behind us. As I approached the approximately fifty-year-old Caucasian male driving the truck, he rolled down his window. He had a look of disbelief on his face.

In a very direct and loud voice I said: "You will not follow an ambulance responding to an emergency call...and if you continue I will make sure you are given a ticket by the police." I pointed my finger at him in a very authoritative way and said: "You got that?!" The man just looked at me with a sheepish smile on his face. He then looked around and noticed the other drivers were all looking at him. I turned, walked back to the Ambulance briskly, and climbed in.

Smiling, my partner asked: "What did he say...ha ha?!"

I responded: "Actually he didn't say anything. He just sat there looking rather stunned."

My partner said: "Well, I bet he never expected that to happen... ha ha!"

As I continued driving toward the accident scene I said: "I have been wanting to do that since I began doing this job, but we never can because we are always responding to a call. This is the first time I have been able to without delaying our response as it was a routine call."

When we arrived at the MVI, my partner and I checked out the three people standing on the roadway and they all declined assessment and treatment.

As we departed the scene, my partner, still smiling, said: "Do you want a coffee Luciano?" I replied: "Sounds like a perfect plan. Let's do that. Hopefully we won't get another call until we do. Could use one."

Brought back to life

It was a typical busy day in the Lower Mainland. It was a non-stop day and we were only half way through our twelve-hour shift. We had been given various calls and some were cancelled due to there being closer cars; this happens often on busy days. We were just on our way to a Code 3 call that would have taken us approximately eight to ten minutes.

Dispatch: "23A2."

My partner replied: "23A2."

Dispatch: "Cancel previous. Have a call you are all over...dropping it on your CAD." "Blip...blip...blip..." The CAD made noise as the screen flashed with the new information on the new call.

I turned the CAD and looked at the call. As I read it I spoke out loud, so my partner could hear the call as he drove. "Code 3 for an OD (overdose). This call is only two blocks away...you will have to do a U-turn to get around this median just ahead. I will get the exact location...give me a sec?"

My partner replied: "OK...so just do a U-turn up here?"

I replied: "Yes, here is good."

I pulled up the mapping screen on the CAD and the call was at a motel just two blocks away.

After we turned around I said: "See that motel just up on the right? That is where we are going to turn."

My partner replied: "Yes I see it."

We pulled in and noticed a female laying supine just underneath the covered area of the walkway outside the motel. A younger male was standing nearby; he began waving and frantically motioning to us as we approached.

After we stopped, I pressed the 'On Scene' button on the CAD. I proceeded to back of Amb and grabbed the jump bag and portable suction; simultaneously, my partner grabbed the O2 tank that is mounted on the back of the door.

I proceeded toward the woman on the sidewalk. As I approached, the twenty-something-year-old male moved toward me. The man spoke: "She went down after we did a hit."

I replied: "What did she take...and how much?"

He said: "She did heroin...one hit."

I moved to her head: she was ashen pale and had cyanotic lips. I shouted at her: "Can you hear me? I'm a Paramedic." I stimulated her by pinching hard on her trapezius: no response. She was an approximately 18-20-year old Caucasian, dressed well, stylish, and did not look like a drug user. I simultaneously began getting equipment as I asked some questions. "Is she a regular user?"

He replied: "No man...it's her nineteenth birthday, so she wanted to celebrate."

I replied: "Has she taken any other drugs or had any alcohol?"

He replied: "No drugs, and only a few beers before we did the hit."

"How many is 'a few' beers?"

My partner beside me now was already getting the O2 ready. I grabbed the pulse oximeter from the kit and placed it on her finger; it read 88%. I quickly pulled the BVM out of the kit and grabbed the OPAs. I measured and inserted a Yellow OPA, positioned her head, placed the BVM mask on her face, and began to ventilate her.

My partner handed me the O2 tubing and I connected it the end of the reservoir bag. I began to bag her once every 5 seconds.

I looked at the O2 Sat monitor and her oxygen saturation was 98% now.

I thought to myself: "Good."

My partner said: "Do you want an IV?"

I replied: "Yeah maybe. Trying to decide if we should narc her here or back in the car...can you grab a quick sugar please?"

My partner replied: "No problem."

Just then the FD pulled up.

Three firemen approached and asked what we needed.

I said: "Can you grab the cot please?" The Captain replied: "Did you want the clam?"

I replied: "No, just the cot will do...thanks. Can one of you take over bagging please?"

Just then my partner said: "Sugar is 5.5."

I replied: "Great. I'm going to draw up the Narcan if you want to get the cot ready."

My partner replied: "Will do. I'll hang a line in the back of the car too."

"Sounds good," I said.

I drew up 2cc (0.8mg) of Narcan to in a 3cc syringe and administered it in the patient's arm in a subcutaneous injection. One of the firefighters said: "The cot is ready."

I replied: "Great. Let's fore-and-aft her to the cot after we give her two more vents."

The firefighter who was bagging gave two slow vents before we moved her. We all worked as a team to get the young woman on the cot. As soon as we finished, I began bagging her again. Before we were able to load her into the Ambulance she began to gag on the OPA I had inserted.

'The Narcan is beginning to work,' I thought.

I removed the OPA and I shouted at her as I gave her a painful sternal rub. "Open your eyes...I'm a Paramedic. We are here to help you." The hearing is the first and last sense to function when unconscious, so announcing who we are lets the person know where they are or who is touching them so they will not panic when they regain consciousness.

I asked the man: "What is her name?"

He replied: "Ashley."

I shouted again: "Ashley, my name is Luke. I'm a Paramedic. We are here to help you." (I will often use 'Luke' as my alias, as my full name, Luciano, is too difficult for people to understand.)

Ashely began to open her eyes now and groan a bit.

I said to my partner: "Let's load her into the car."

He replied: "OK, sounds good."

We loaded her into the car, took a set of vitals, and started an IV. Soon, she was able to speak and began apologizing over and over.

"I'm so sorry," Ashley said. "I'm sorry, I didn't mean to do this. I'm so embarrassed."

I replied: "It's OK, just glad we got to you in time. You were blue and barely breathing when we got to you."

Ashely said: "I'm so sorry, it was my birthday. I have not used any in over a year."

I replied: "I know, your friend told me. It's OK, you will be OK now. We are going to take you to the hospital so you can be monitored, OK?"

She replied: "Yes, OK, I'm so sorry."

My partner called from the driver's seat now: "You good to go?"

I replied: "Yes, routine is fine, thanks."

We headed toward the local hospital, which was only a short eight-minute drive away.

After speaking to the Triage nurse and handing the patient over, I headed out to the car where my partner was just finishing making up the cot. As I approached he said: "Wow, there is some strong heroin on the street this week, that is the fourth OD I have heard about in the last two days."

I replied: "Yes, no kidding. Seems like every crew out this way is doing at least one per couple days...I think I need a coffee."

My partner replied: "Sure, sounds good. Could use a few minutes before the next call."

I replied: "OK let's see if we can sneak to the Starbucks down the road before we clear. I would like to get a few sips in before the next call."

My partner replied: "Let's do it."

Spear in the leg

The day was a beautiful sunny day. I was working near the ocean this shift. We were just driving from cross-covering another community when the CAD sounded.

"Blip...blip...blip."

I was attending today, so I turned the CAD toward me and read the screen:

- Code 3
- 14yo female with a spear embedded in the leg, on the beach
- Auto launch initiated
- Pt Conscious and breathing
- Fire Department reponding

Dispatch came over the radio: "43V, be advised that auto launch has be initiated and 99T will be departing the airport."

My partner replied: "43V – 10-4."

I said to my partner: "We have a fourteen-year-old with a spear embedded in her leg on Rocky beach...it's Code 3."

She replied: "Really? Wow."

My partner activated the lights and siren as sped toward the beach that was at least fourteen minutes from our location. I called Dispatch on the cell phone for more information. The dispatcher advised that the girl had been boogie-boarding and the anchor pulled out, embedding in her leg.

When we arrived at the beach, there were a lot of people milling about, but nobody was waving us in as we expected; they just stood there looking at us. It always amazes me when people just stare at us like we are aliens that just arrived.

I said to my partner: "Hey I'm just going to get out and figure out where the patient is, since nobody is waving us in."

She replied: "OK, I'm going to speak to Fire and find out if they have an LZ set up yet."

"Sounds good."

I then walked toward a log fence line and asked a few people if they knew who had called us. Suddenly, a woman approached me with a look of panic in her eyes. "She is on the beach, down over here," she said.

I replied: "OK, I will get my kit. Will need you to lead us down, OK?"

"OK."

I headed back to the car, spoke to my partner about what I had found out, and then grabbed the kit and O2 out of the car. We proceeded down on foot to the beach. We could see the patient in the distance, near the water's edge.

When we arrived, Fire was on scene and began with a verbal report as I moved to check the injured leg. I noticed a large white trauma dressing over the mid-thigh area.

Fire: "So this is Melissa. She is 14, and was boogie-boarding with that anchor in" — pointing to the two-foot spike laying on the sand — "and it pulled out, came right back at her, and embedded in her leg."

"Thanks," I replied, and knelt down to Meliss.

"Hi Melissa, my name is Luc. I'm a Paramedic. How are you feeling right now?"

Melissa replied: "My leg is hurting, but otherwise not too bad."

I said: "OK, well we are going to get you off the beach and up to the Ambulance. I just want to take a look at the wound, OK?"

Melissa replied: "OK, but I don't want to look."

"You don't have to look," I replied.

I pulled away the dressing and saw a gaping wound to the inner thigh. It was approximately ten centimetres long and had cut through the full thickness of her flesh; it looked like it was down to bone. It was not bleeding though, so I knew it had not hit any vital blood vessels. I re-dressed the wound with a clean dressing and applied a trauma strap. Just then, the FD arrived with a basket stretcher. We loaded the girl into the stretcher and began walking toward our Ambulance parked at the edge of the parking lot. We could hear the helicopter approaching in the distance as we moved her toward the shoreline.

When we arrived at the Ambulance, the main cot had already been prepared with a #9 to ready her for transport in the helicopter. The helo landed shortly thereafter, and the airflight paramedics arrived for handover.

The airflight paramedic walked up with a smile on his face: "Hi guys what do we have?" I replied: "This is Melissa. She is 14, was out wakeboarding, and an anchor that had been placed on shore pulled out and stabbed her in the right thigh. It is down to the femur but not bleeding. Looks like it missed the artery."

Airflight paramedic: "OK, let's get her loaded up and take her to Children's Hospital." We all helped get her loaded into the medical evac helicopter and watched it take off. It's always exciting for the public when a helicopter lands, especially if it is a medi-vac.

Foot Crushed

It was a typical dayshift working in a town in the greater Vancouver area. I had a good partner and we were steady as usual, which is typical when there are not enough cars to cover the calls coming in. I was attending, and we had just been sent on yet another cross coverage to the nearby town. This was our second trip to this cross-coverage area. Earlier we had been sent to the area and on the way I had asked my partner if we could stop by and look at a guitar I was thinking of buying from Craigslist. He had no problem with it and happened to be an avid guitar player himself. We had made it to the residence and after my partner 'Scott' looked the guitar over, I bought it. I placed it in the back of the Ambulance, tucked in behind our rear chair we referred to 'the captain's chair.' We had returned to our station and had just sat down when the phone rang, and we were sent back to the cross coverage area.

Scott said: "Well, looks like it is going to be one of those days...and they say we are not short of resources...but hey we just don't know the bigger picture."

I replied: "Right, the bigger picture...ha ha they should be out here, so by the time we get to the cross coverage point there will be no ambulances covering this community or we will be ten to fifteen minutes Code 3 to get back...brilliant!"

As we approached the cross-coverage area, a call came in; the CAD sounded: "Blip...blip...blip." I spun the CAD toward me as I read the call details. It was a routine call for an ankle injury at an industrial work site. I pushed the 'En Route' button and said to Scott: "Looks like we have a call just ahead at the big bakery. Should be there in less than five minutes."

Scott replied: "Great, we will actually have a great response time for a change."

"No kidding," I said.

As we approached the turn, the radio squawked: "87A1 cancel the last and take instead."

The CAD sounded: "Blip...blip...blip."

- Code 3 for a fall off of a balcony > than 10ft
- 87yo Pt is unconscious
- FD is responding

Dispatch called on the radio: "87A2 I just dropped a Code 3 call on your CAD."

I hit the 'En Route' button as we drove past the entrance road to the bakery. Scott lit up the Ambulance and turned on the siren. It was a dry day, with an overcast sky and moderate traffic. We were approximately nine minutes away from the call, driving Code 3.

Approximately one minute later, the CAD squawked again: "Blip...blip...blip."

Dispatch: "Sorry guys, have to take you off this call. Just dropped a new call on your CAD."

I looked at the CAD and read the new call information:

- Code 3 for SOB 30 yo female
- History of anxiety
- FD responding

I looked at the call in disbelief.

"You won't believe this Scott! We are being cancelled from a fall off a balcony. These f**king call-takers!! They are morons! So, a short-of-breath thirty-year-old with a history of anxiety is higher acuity than a fall off of a balcony?"

Scott just shook his head and replied: "Well, you should be used to this by now. Doesn't make sense."

I said: "I know I should — it happens all the time — but I just can't get used to moronic stupidity! The MPDS (Medical Priority Dispatch System) has a lot of flaws and if the person taking the call has never worked the streets and is a paramedic, how can they possibly ask the right questions?"

We were just approaching the bridge that moves us into the next community where the call was located when Dispatch called on the radio.

Dispatch: "87A1, cancel that last. I will just get you to do some coverage for now."

Scott turned off the emergency equipment and grabbed the mike and replied: "10-4."

Scott said, "Well, looks like we are not needed...yet again!"

I replied: "Yeah, and I wonder what is happening with that ankle injury call were sent to originally. Guess it must be a minor sprain or something and they just need transport. They should just put him into a company truck if it is that minor."

Scott replied: "No kidding. Well, until then, we chill."

Scott parked at a dead-end road near the bridge. After parking, he got out and went to the back of the Amb; when he reappeared, he had the guitar I had bought earlier that morning.

I looked over at him and began to chuckle. "Are you going to serenade me with something...ha ha! This is priceless, we get cancelled off of a routine call and two Code 3 calls and now we are sitting on coverage while you play the guitar."

Scott replied: "Well, why not? I'll tune it up for you."

I said: "Sounds good to me, maybe you can give me a few pointers about playing, I'm looking forward to starting to learn to play."

We sat and waited at cross coverage as Scott played and tuned my guitar. After about thirty minutes, the CAD sounded: "Blip...blip...blip."

I looked at the CAD and on it was the original call for the ankle injury with some new details:

- Blood seeping from boot
- FD dispatched due to delay in ambulance.

I said, "OK, you won't believe this. Remember that ankle injury? Well, they have sent Fire there because of a delay in response and we have been sitting here for over half an hour while you play the guitar, and we are only five minutes away from this call. What is wrong with our dispatcher today?...Morons!!"

Scott replied: "We don't know the bigger picture remember?!!"

Scott left the cab to put the guitar back in the case and tucked it in again behind the captain's chair in the back of the Ambulance.

We arrived at the bakery in less than six minutes, and a staff member was outside flagging us down. As we opened the back doors of the Ambulance, the staff member approached us and said: "The employee is in the warehouse with the first aid attendant. The Fire Department are also with him."

I replied: "Do you know what happened?"

The staffer replied: "He got injured with his forklift."

My mind began to race a bit: this was obviously more than a sprained ankle.

We loaded the kit, O2, Entonox, pillow splint and trauma straps onto the cot and wheeled it into the building. The staff member led us to an open area with a forklift nearby. The Fire Department crew was with the patient who was laying on the ground, supported by another colleague, and had an oxygen mask on. As I approached, I could see blood seeping out of his boot, with a small five-centimetre pool on the concrete floor.

I knelt down by the patient and asked: "What happened?"

Patient replied: "I was driving my forklift and it approached that other forklift as I was turning, I put my foot out to push off the other forklift and my foot was crushed in between them." Surprised by this story, I looked at the forklifts again. They appeared to be 10,000-pound warehouse forklifts. I thought to myself, 'How in the world did he think he was going to stop the forklift from hitting the other one with his foot?...Wow.'

Scott had connected the O2 sat monitor on the patient and it read '98%.'

Scott said: "Hey do you still want the O2 on?"

I replied: "No, let's grab a set of vitals and I am going to check him out. I will need your help to remove his boot in a few minutes."

Scott replied: "Sounds good."

The Fire Captain said: "Is there anything you want my guys to do?"
I replied: "If you can have one of your guys stabilize the foot until I get a chance to examine it, that would be great."

The Fire Captain directed one of his crew to hold the foot and I continued with my assessment of the patient.

I said to the patient: "How did you get where you are?"

Patient: "After my foot was squished between the forklifts I landed here." The Industrial First Aid attendant confirmed that is where he found the patient.

Continuing my assessment, I asked, "Did you hit your head, or lose consciousness?" As I questioned him, I felt his head and neck area.

Patient: "No."

Me: "Are you hurt anyplace else other than your foot?"

Patient: "No."

Me: "OK, I am going to check from your pelvis down to your foot. Let me know if you have any pain, tenderness or numbness anyplace as I do so, OK?"

Patient: "OK."

I proceeded to do a modified primary exam and worked my way down to his injured foot. I had Scott help me as we cut and removed his boot and sock. When his foot was exposed, I was a bit shocked by what I saw, considering how this call was delayed and the lack of urgency given. There was an open wound the size of a toonie on the top of his foot, and obvious crushing had occurred. I checked distal pulses and circulation to the foot – all were present. We began to dress the foot and prepare it for the pillow splint.

I said to the patient, "On a scale of 0-10 with 0 being no pain and 10 being severe pain, what would you rate your pain in your foot?"

Patient: "I would give it a 7 or 8, but I have a pretty good pain tolerance."

I replied: "OK, and I would say yes you do as I have been surprised how well you have been tolerating this pain since we have been here."

Patient: "Well, I was in the military and learned to tough it out."

I offered to give him Entonox and he agreed. So, Scott mixed the gas for me (the tank is tipped side to side a minimum of three times as it contains 50% Oxygen mixed with 50% nitrous oxide) and prepped the regulator. The gas is administered by the patient and they take as much as needed with use of a bite stick they suck on through a demand regulator. We packaged the patient and, with the help of the Fire Department, loaded him onto the cot and wheeled him out to the Ambulance.

After arriving at the local hospital fifteen minutes away and giving triage to the nurse, the patient was transferred to a bed. The ER doctor came in to the cast room when we transferred the patient and was amazed at the extent of the injury and suspected he would have to be transferred to orthotics at a higher acuity hospital in the area.

A few hours later, I checked in with the ER doctor and asked to see the x-ray. The foot was badly fractured with multiple breaks to the metatarsals. The ER doctor told me that the patient would be transferred out the following day. The next day, we were the crew that transferred the patient to orthotics in the other hospital.

Due to the delay in the call, I spoke to my supervisor about a call review on this call, as it was unnecessarily delayed – the supervisor agreed.

Approximately a month later I just happened to be in that higher level of care hospital and this patient happened to be wheeled past. He had multiple pins sticking out of his foot and had been in the hospital for over a month. It was a strong reminder of how getting accurate call information should have upgraded this call to 'Code 3' at the time. Fortunately, his injury was not limb-threatening or he could have lost his foot due to lack of blood flow.

CPR on the alive guy

It was a busy day and we had a three-man crew due to one of the paramedics being on a return-to-work detail. We had just cleared the hospital and our CAD sounded — "Blip...blip...blip" — as the call came across the screen:

- Code 3 for an unconscious OD
- FD responding

Dispatch called: "75A2...ALS not available. It's just you and the Fire."

I replied: "75A2 10-4."

We arrived at a residence, and a Caucasian woman was standing in the driveway. I parked and headed in as Don (the return-to-work paramedic) grabbed the kit and my regular partner (Mark), who was in the back, grabbed the O2 from the back door. We headed toward the woman standing in the driveway.

As we approached, I said to the woman, "Who are we here for?"

The woman replied: "It's my son. He took heroin."

Don followed in behind the woman and I was close behind. I did not notice Mark, who had been in the back of the ambulance, and just assumed he was a few steps behind us. We walked into a basement room that was well-lit. As we walked around the corner, we could see a man's legs laying on the floor. Don rounded the corner first.

Suddenly, Don said in an intense manner: "Why are you doing CPR on someone who is alive?...Stop!" I rounded the corner just as he was saying this and could see an adult woman doing chest compressions on a Caucasian male on the floor. His eyes were open, and it looked like he was trying to say something. The woman who was doing chest compressions stopped and looked up at Don.

The woman said: "You want me to stop? Really?"

Don replied: "Yes, I can see he is alive."

The woman paused for a moment and looked like she wanted to go back onto the chest, then hesitated and just stayed there.

I moved in behind her. "Can you move out of the way please?" I asked.

She moved away from the patient, who appeared to be a twenty-year-old Caucasian male. His chest was bare and he was wearing blue jeans. His eyes were still open and he was looking around. (Sometimes people in cardiac arrest will have their eyes open but they will usually be glazed over and milky in color, a sign of impending death). This man's eyes were clearly bright and full of life he had good color in his face and was not cyanotic.

As Don began to get a history I moved in and checked the patient's radial pulse. It was present; he was breathing slowly but effectively at a rate of 12 breaths per minute.

Don said: "Let's get a non-rebreather on him."

Mark, who had brought in the O2, pulled out a mask and handed it to me, as I was closer to the patient. Don, who now had gotten a history, learned that the woman doing compressions earlier was the patient's sister.

Don asked: "So, do you know how much he used?"

The sister replied: "We think he used a point?"

Just then, the patient began to make some moaning noises.

Don shouted at him: "Hey Jordan (patients name)!" The patient moaned again, and his eyes flickered open for a minute.

I yelled at the patient: "Jordan, open your eyes! We are paramedics. We are here to help you!"

The patient opened his eyes slightly and moaned again and said: "My chest hurts."

I think Don and I looked at each other simultaneously with the look of 'I guess your chest hurts, your sister just did chest compressions on you.'

We continued our assessment, auscultated his chest for air entry to see if any ribs punctured his chest wall. Everything seemed intact. Being a young man, his chest was very elastic and able to withstand more than someone who was older, I thought.

Don said: "OK Jordan, we have to take you to the hospital."

Jordan replied: "I'm not going to the hospital I am fine."

Don said: "You sister did chest compressions on your chest you need an assessment and possibly a chest x-ray."

Jordan replied: "Well, I am not going," and slowly got up and walked out of the room.

Jordan's sister went after him and pleaded with him to go with us. Both Don and I also tried to convince him to go to the hospital. Jordan would have nothing of it. We finally were forced to have him sign a release, witnessed by his sister. We could not force him to go.

We packed our equipment and left the residence.

DOA

The day was a normal busy day — call after call with no chance to even grab a coffee. I had a student this block (a row of four shifts), as I was a preceptor. It was raining today, and the student was in the back of the Ambulance.

The CAD suddenly sounded: "Blip...blip...blip." I looked at the screen and read what it said:

- Code 3, police not on scene
- Suspected Code 4
- Fire Dept responding

I said to my partner: "Looks like we are going to a dead guy."

My partner, Don, replied: "Oh really?...Where is it?"

I replied: "I will guide you in...continue on here and turn left in a few blocks."

Don replied: "Sure, OK."

I called back to my student: "Erica, have you ever seen a dead body before?"

Erica replied: "No...but I'm not worried about it."

I replied: "OK...well what's going to happen is I will go in first, then my partner. We will verify death. It's considered a crime scene by the police until proven otherwise, so careful where you step and don't touch or pick up anything. Depending on the condition of the body, I will come out and get you if you want to view it."

Erica replied: "OK...I'm not afraid to see a dead body."

I replied: "Good to know."

It only took us approximately six minutes to get to the call.

When we arrived, I pushed the "On Scene" button. We could see two police cars outside of a low-income apartment building.

As we got out of the Amb, I grabbed the jump-bag and my stethoscope. while my partner grabbed the O2 and AED. I approached a male police officer and he began to tell me that the landlord gained access when the resident had not been heard from for days and a smell began emitting from the apartment. The police had just arrived on scene and had not entered the residence yet.

We headed into the building with the police in the lead. We could hear sirens in the distance, most likely the fire department. As we proceeded down the dimly lit hallway and got closer to the door, I could smell the unmistakable smell of a rotting corpse. The door was unlocked as I entered the residence behind the two police officers.

The smell was very strong now. One of the officers remarked: "Right here, in the bathroom." I entered the bathroom and saw a Caucasian man completely naked and submerged except for his face in a bathtub full of water. I was clear that he had been there for a number of days. I could see post-mortem lividity on the sides of his body, and he was bloating from the gases that occur after a person dies. It was not a pleasant sight.

I exited the bathroom and walked up to my partner, Don. "Well, he is definitely dead."

Don replied: "I'm taking it you don't have to do a pulse check or check for signs of life?"

I replied: "Definitely not, not in this case."

Don entered the bathroom, stayed a few moments, then exited. Upon exiting, he exclaimed: "Nope, definitely dead!"

The fire department arrived on scene with their equipment (jumpbag O2 and AED). I noticed the Fire Captain and said: "We are all good Cap, this guy is gone."

The Captain said: "OK, do you guys need us for anything?"

I replied: "No we are good, thanks." The fire department then left the scene.

Erica appeared, standing at the doorway. I could tell she wanted to see the guy in the tub. "Do you want to see the body?" I asked.

Erica replied somewhat eagerly: "Yes I do!"

I replied: "OK, but I want to tell you something...It's not a pleasant sight, so be prepared OK?"

Erica replied: "OK...I'm not worried."

Erica proceeded to enter the bathroom, stayed a few minutes, then exited. I looked at her face for any unusual emotion or expression, but she looked fine.

I asked the police if they needed a copy of our patient care report and they told me they did. I said I would write it up in the Ambulance and give them a copy before we left. Don, Erica, and I left the apartment and proceeded to the Ambulance. I completed my patient care report and gave it to one of the other officers before we cleared.

I called back to Erica: "So how was your first dead body experience?"

Erica replied: "I'm fine. Guess I wanted to know how I would feel about seeing it."

I replied: "Well that one was kinda bad visually and the smell, so if you are OK with that, most others are not as bad. The thing is, you may experience some unusual feeling about it later today, tomorrow, or next week. Just do some self-checks; make sure you are OK with what you saw and smelled. We have resources if it begins to bother you."

Erica replied: "OK thanks. I'm sure I will be OK, but appreciate knowing that."

Don said: "Yeah, you don't have to pretend you are tough. It can bother anyone, or it may not at all. Everyone is different."

Erica replied: "Sure, OK."

I hit 'Clear' on the CAD and we departed the scene.

Slipped on Carpet

It was another busy night, and I was attending. We had just cleared a call when our CAD sounded: "Blip...blip...blip." My partner looked at the CAD and exclaimed,: "Great...yet another urgent call requiring an ambulance! Fourteen-year-old back pain."

I replied: "Hmmm great! This should be interesting...I bet there are cars in the driveway and people home to drive the kid to the hospital." My partner noted the address; it was about fifteen minutes away, routine.

We arrived at a very large, new home with three cars in the driveway. "I knew it!" I said. "Now let's see if there is anyone to drive them." My partner backed in the driveway and I said: "Let's check this out, see what we have. I will just bring the kit for now."

We were met at the door by an East Indian man in his late 50s. I said: "Who are we here to see sir?"

He replied: "Oh, my son he is upstairs."

I said: "OK, we will follow you."

M partner and I followed the man to an upper bedroom. The house was huge, like a mansion. When we arrived at the upper bedroom, there were six other family members in the room, from younger kids to grandparents. The man motioned to a younger boy sitting on the carpet. There were three carpeted steps that led to an elevated bed in the room.

I approached him and said: "Hi, are we here to see you?"

He replied: "Yes."

I said: "So what happened?"

He replied: "I was walking down the steps, slipped and landed on my back."

I said: "OK, are you hurt?"

He replied: "My back is sore."

"OK, any pain in your neck?" I asked, as I gently palpated his neck from the base to the upper thoracic area of his spine.

He replied: "No."

I continued with my assessment and after determining that he had minor pain in his lower back he was assisted to stand. He indicated he had some minor back pain — two out of ten on the pain scale.

I turned to the father and said: "It looks like a muscular strain. I cannot do extensive tests here. Do you want us to transport him to the hospital?"

The man replied: "Yes."

I turned to the fourteen-year-old boy and said: "OK let's go. Get your shoes on the way out and we will take you to the hospital to get you checked out by a doctor.

Before leaving the home, I turned to the father and said: "Sir, is there anyone going to follow us to the hospital?" He replied: "Yes, we will follow. Are you going to Normand hospital?" "Yes," I replied.

The boy was led to the Ambulance and asked to sit in one of our high-backed chairs that we often refer to as the 'captain's chair.' My partner hopped in and we departed routine to Normand hospital. The boy was walked to a minor treatment and assessment area after being triaged and sat in the waiting room with his family that drove to the hospital.

When we got back in the Ambulance, my partner said: "We, that was a waste of time...What, have they never seen their son slip on the carpet before?...Geeez what a waste of the system."

I replied: "Yup...three cars in the driveway and they call an ambulance for a back strain from a slip on the carpet...brilliant!"

Handcuffs

We were working a night shift, and my regular partner for the block had booked off sick so was working with another irreg. It was my drive night and we were just sitting at cross coverage when a call came in: "Blip...blip...blip."

My partner (Jack) looked at the CAD: "Oh, a nine-year-old in handcuffs with circulation cut off."

I replied: "Really? So are the Code 5s coming on this?...Ha ha."

Jack said: "Nope...not on the CAD. The Code 6s are not coming either."

I spun the CAD toward me and read the call:
- Location: 4578 No place Drive Big town
- Response: Code 2
- Type: 1C4
- Radio: Anytown EHS – 4
- Call Source: Person at scene
- Units: 29A2
- Remarks: 9yo male, in handcuffs, circulation being cut off

I said: "So, we are responding to a nine-year-old in handcuffs and the police are not attending...brilliant call-taking once again! So how are we supposed to remove the handcuffs? I just happen to carry a hand-cuff key because of my previous careers, but they don't know that. The police should have been on this call before we were even called. Bunch of morons!!"

Jack replied: "No kidding, and without Fire to cut them off, what are we supposed to do?"

I said: "Well, when we get closer maybe we should ask for the police and or Fire to respond...Still can't believe they are sending a Paramedic crew to a call with a patient handcuffed knowing we have no way of removing them…I mean really!!"

We continued on, as it was a fair distance away. When we got within ten minutes of the call, Jack said; "I'm going to call Dispatch and ask for them to send Fire, in case we need them to cut the cuffs off." He grabbed the cell phone and spoke to Dispatch. After he hung up he said: "OK, they said Fire won't respond unless we request that we need them."

I replied: "Ha ha, great…Well, guess we will just figure it out when we get there. They might not be standard handcuffs, so my key won't work, but if they are I will just remove them and go from there. I think I will call on the air to see if they are going to send the 5s." A few moments later I grabbed the mike and spoke into it: "29 Alpha 2."

Dispatch: "29A2."

I replied: "29A2…just wondering if the 5s are on this call?"

Dispatch: "No the 5s are not indicated."

I replied: "Well, just wondering since the patient is in handcuffs… Don't worry we will figure it out."

I said to Jack. "I just can't believe it…ha ha."

We heard the radio squawk: "29A2, the Code 6 said they are responding."

I grabbed the mike and replied: "10-4."

We arrived a few minutes later beside a newer home in a very nice peaceful suburban neighbourhood. It was quiet as it was just after midnight. I parked on the roadway, turned on my four-way flashers, and when we exited the Amb we noticed a young woman standing outside the house on the lighted porch. I moved toward the house as my partner grabbed the kit. As I approached I said: "Hi, who are we here to see?"

She replied: "Oh…it's my brother, he is inside. I will lead you in."

I said: "Perfect, thanks."

I followed her in, with Jack a few steps behind us. We walked into the living room and there were three young boys. One was sitting on the couch with silver handcuffs around his wrists. I said to the boy with handcuffs: "So, how did this happen?"

The boy replied: "Well..." — laughing a bit — "I put these handcuffs on and did not know where the key is."

With a smile, I said: "Well, that was not a good idea. OK, let me take a look."

The boy held his hands up and I looked at the handcuffs. They were a cheap pot metal and did not have a standard (real) handcuff keyhole.

I turned to my partner: "Well, looks like my key won't work. I am going to go out to the car and see if we have a set of small bolt cutters. Some of the cars in remote areas used to have them. I did not see a set in the car, but will take a look until Fire arrives."

Jack replied: "OK, sounds good."

I went outside looked through the car and could not find them. Just then, a fire pumper truck pulled up, the stopped beside me. I said: "Hey guys, thanks. We are going to need bolt cutters to cut off the cuffs."

The fire truck driver said: "OK, just going to pull up there and we will be right in."

I led the way inside and one of the firemen had bolt cutters with him. It only took a few snips and the handcuffs were off. Jack took a look at the boy's wrist and there were some marks but no circulation impairment.

The fire crew left the scene. We had the boy sign our paperwork (saying that he did not want to go to hospital) and had his older sister witness it. We left the house and after getting back into the Amb, Jack and I just looked at each other and at the same time said: "OK, that was interesting." We both started to laugh.

Cut Finger

I was working a night shift. We were at the station which was unusual for this area. The hotline rang, and the dispatcher told me there was a call on the CAD.

We headed out to the bay and climbed in. I spun the CAD and read the call:

- Code 3 for possible major hemorrhage/life threatening
- 23 yo male cut his finger with an exacto knife

I said to my partner: "OK, really...Code 3 for major hemorrhage from a cut finger!! Seriously?! The guy could cut his finger off and would not bleed out for a while. Last time I checked, there are no arteries in the finger...Stupid call takers....geez."

My partner spun the CAD and looked at it and said: "Well just another moronic call...Can't believe people call ambulances for this. This should be interesting."

My partner headed out on the street. Traffic was fairly light and the call was less than four minutes away. He didn't activate the emergency equipment on the Ambulance, and I said nothing, as I agreed this call should not have been coded 'major hemorrhage/life threatening.'

We pulled up to a residence and as we stopped and activated the side-scene lights, a man and woman began approaching the Ambulance on foot. The man was holding his hand with a towel. I got out and approached them.

"Hi, are we here for you?" I asked.

The man replied: "Yes, I cut my hand with an exacto knife...think I need stitches. It's pretty deep."

I replied: "OK, let's get you inside the Ambulance and take a look."

We entered though the side door and my student continued to ask questions. "What were you doing?"

Patient: "I'm an upholstery installer but was working on my own car. Knife slipped and cut down to bone I think. It was bleeding a lot initially."

We exposed the wound. By this point, the bleeding had virtually stopped was just oozing out slowly from a clean laceration at the index finger tip. We cleaned the wound with wound cleaner, covered it in clean telfa, and wrapped it in gauze.

The patient said: "I was going to get my girlfriend to drive me, but she can't drive standard. I have cut my fingers a few times and needed stitches."

The girlfriend, who was in the Ambulance, replied: "Yeah, I guess I could have borrowed the landlord's truck and driven you?"

The patient replied: "Yeah, I guess you could have. Maybe you can follow us to the hospital so I have a drive home?"

Girlfriend: "OK, I will ask him after you leave."

I said "OK, let's run you up to the hospital. Certainly looks like you need some sutures."

We brought the patient to the hospital and he was walked to a minor treatment area to await sutures. After we got back into the Ambulance my partner said: "You think they would have thought to borrow the landlord's truck before they called 911. Seriously how do people cope? That would never have happened in the rural areas."

I replied: "Yes, I agree...but I am still pissed that the moronic call takers assigned that as a 'Code 3' call."

Pepper Spray

On a normal busy night, I had a student with us and we were just driving back to the station from dropping our last patient off in the hospital when the CAD sounded: "Blip...blip...blip."

I looked at the CAD; it read:

- Location: 711
- Response: Code 2
- Type: Post Assault/Robbery
- Call source: Police
- Units: 77A1
- Remarks:
- Police on scene
- Male possible pepper sprayed

I yelled back to my student: "Looks like you get to treat a pepper spray."

The student replied: "Cool."

My partner replied: "Great...when are we going to get some interesting calls? This block has been so boring."

When we arrived, we could see two police cars in the parking lot and noticed a man against the wall near the entrance. He was pacing and holding his face, while talking to the police. I said to the student: "We will need a few IV bags and some bottles of saline as well as the baby shampoo." We use baby shampoo as it does not sting the eyes and is needed to remove the sticky pepper spray from the skin.

We exited the Ambulance and brought our supplies over to the patient. One of the RCMP officers approached us and said "So this guy was bear-sprayed in the face, just post a robbery at this store. Looks like wrong place wrong time." A late 40s early 50s Caucasian man was moving about, holding his face. We walked over and approached the man.

I said: "Sir, my name is Luke (always use a short version of my name, my full name is too difficult for patients to remember anyway). Do you remember what happened?"

The man replied: "Yeah, I was just getting a coffee and leaving and was fucking pepper sprayed. My eyes and face are burning."

I replied: "OK, we will begin flushing out your eyes in a minute. Did you fall on the ground or were you hit by the guys who pepper sprayed you?" The patient replied: "No."

I said: "OK, we are going to flush your eyes to get the pepper spray out."

The man replied: "OK, hurry it's burning like crazy."

I took a 1000ml IV bag of normal saline and cut off the end with my scissors. I said to my student: "OK get in here. You irrigate while I hold his eyes open."

The student said: "OK."

As we began irrigating, I instructed the patient: "Open your eyes. Blink blink blink..."

Patient replied: "Damn it burns...it's getting worse."

I said: "I know. As the oils start coming out it burns more. We have to keep flushing."

I grabbed the baby shampoo and said: "Open your hands. I have baby shampoo. It will help remove the pepper spray from your skin." I poured some into his hands and said: "Rub this all over your face and head."

We irrigated the man's eyes, alternating with baby shampoo to remove the residue. My partner stood by and watched as the student and I flushed the patient's eyes and poured water over his head so he could scrub his face and head to remove the peppery spray. After approximately fifteen minutes, the man was able to open his eyes without extensive burning.

I said: "Sir, you need to go home and have a shower. Walk directly into the shower with your clothes on and remove them with the water running. They will be contaminated with the pepper spray. Scrub from head to toe with this baby shampoo and remove all the oils from your skin. Once most of the burning has stopped you can exit the shower.

Make sure you launder your clothing separately, so you don't cross-contaminate other clothing...do you understand?"

The patient replied: "Yes, yes I get it."

I asked the police officer if they needed anything else from us and we were released from the scene.

As we left the scene the student said: "Wow there are a lot of pepper spray incidents in this area." My partner replied: "Yeah, it's a fun place to work sometimes...we get all kinds."

239kph

I was working OT on (what was supposed to be) my second day off. I had been cold-called only an hour and a half before the shift at a nearby semi-rural station. It was an afternoon shift from noon until 11:00pm. I had never worked with my part-time partner before and I was attending today. We were having a good shift, except we kept getting tagged with calls in the city as we tried to get back to our area. We were just approaching the freeway and the CAD sounded "Blip...blip...blip." I spun the CAD screen toward me as my partner groaned: "Oh...really!! We are never going to make it back at this rate...ha ha." He was a happy, positive guy, but wanted to get back to the station as much as I did.

I looked at the screen and read the details of the call out loud: "We have a roll-over MVI, high speed, Code 3, in the ditch. On person on scene walking. It's not far from where we are. Just head toward the freeway...it's the next exit." The road was dry, there was no rain, and it was cool out, but not cold, on this spring day in the late afternoon. It was just getting dark as we sped toward the call. The CAD sounded multiple times as we proceeded toward the call, giving us updates on location, number of persons involved, etc.

We took the next off-ramp and proceeded toward the call. Just as we went over the overpass, a fire ladder truck was turning around just ahead of us. We continued around the onramp until we came across a car turned onto its side in the ditch. There was a younger Caucasian male leaning against the police car, talking to an officer.

We parked and I grabbed my high visibility vest from the door and proceeded toward the police car. I approached the man speaking to the officer.

I said: "Is this the driver of the car?"

The officer replied: "Yes."

I said: "I have to speak to him immediately regarding the crash." The officer moved away from the man, who was leaning against the hood of the car. I looked down and he was not wearing shoes. He was only wearing a t-shirt and jeans. He was turning his head about freely and had a slight dazed look about him.

I said: "Were you the driver of the car?"

He replied: "Yes sir."

I said: "Did you get out of the car yourself?"

He replied: "Yes...I can still talk to the officer."

I said: "The officer can talk to you later. I need to do an assessment on you now. Do you have any pain anyplace?"

Patient replied: "Yeah, I have pain in my back."

I exposed his back and said: "Where is the pain? Show me."

The patient replied; "It's right here." He moved his hands around the mid and lower back area. I looked and there was no broken skin, no abrasions or swelling.

I said: "Do you have any pain in your head or neck?"

Patient replied: "No."

I said: "Did you lose consciousness?"

Patient: "No...I'm really sorry man."

I said: "It's OK...OK we are going to check you out further in the back of the Ambulance. You were the only one in the car?"

Patient: "Yes sir."

I said: "What is your name?"

The patient replied: "Tylor."

I replied: "OK Tylor, my name is Luke. We are going to check you out a bit more in the back of the Ambulance."

As I began walking the patient to the Ambulance, my partner approached us. He had already opened the side door of the Ambulance.

My partner said: "I checked the car there is nobody else in it." I replied: "Perfect. We are just going to check him out in the back of the car, do vitals, etc."

My partner nodded, and went ahead and opened the bed pack up before we entered. The patient stepped up into the Ambulance. We had him lay on the cot, and I obtained his BP (134/76), pulse rate (74 Regular), O2 sats (95%), and breathing rate (18 per minute). Everything was in normal limits. I did a complete head to toe examination, including auscultating his chest for breath sounds. His only complaint was pain in his mid-back down to his lower back.

I said: "Do you remember everything that happened?"

Tylor replied: "I was on the phone with my mom. We had an argument. I was on the way to the office, and that is the last thing I remember."

I said: "Do you remember driving off the road?"

Tylor replied: "No."

I said: "Do you remember getting out of the car?"

Tylor replied: "No...ahhh I am so sorry."

I said: "Do you know what day it is...your birthday?"

Tylor replied; "It's.....Monday, Sept 12, 1979."

I said: "OK, so the only thing bothering you is your back at this time?"

Tylor replied: "Yes...hurts."

I turned to my partner and said: "I'm going to take a look at the car. I want to get a closer look at the mechanism."

My partner replied: "Do you want me to take a look at the car?"

I replied: "No thanks, I want to see the car. If you could stay with the patient, I will be right back."

My partner said: "No problem."

I excited the Ambulance and walked toward the car, flashlight out. One of the firefighters on scene said: "Are you looking for his wallet?"

I replied: "Ah, no, I am just checking out the car for mechanism."

I went over to the embankment as the firefighter followed me. I shined my flashlight inside the car. All the airbags were deployed: driver's, curtain, side, knee. There was no broken glass inside the car. The seatbelt was intact and released from the clip. The firefighter said: "His wallet is on the bottom, see?" as he shined his flashlight inside the car. I looked and saw the wallet laying on the passenger side window of the car, which was resting on its side.

The firefighter said: "Do you want to try to get the wallet?"

I said: "Move back a minute." I deployed my knife with the window break on it and popped the sunroof. The glass shattered into small pieces and I noticed the area of the sunroof was covered by a sunshield.

The firefighter said: "Oh, man, it's covered. I can reach in and get it if you hold the door open for me"

I said, "Sure," thinking that it was a good idea if he did it, as he was wearing his turnout gear which would protect him from sharp edges. He was able to grab the wallet and pull it out, and hand it to me. "Great, thanks," I said.

As I walked back toward the edge of the road, I jumped over a muddy area of the embankment. One of the other firefighters said: "This car came from that off-ramp not this one" (as he pointed to an off-ramp, a few hundred feet away), "and was clocked at 239kph." I looked in that direction and was shocked by hearing this from the firefighter and not the police officer who had been interviewing the patient when we pulled up.

I said: "So the car came from way over there?"

The firefighter replied: "Yes."

I walked across the onramp toward the other off-ramp to see if I could see where the tires last made contact with the ground, as the car had cleared a concrete road barrier, three feet high, that guarded the outer side of the onramp we were on. I walked through the grass and muddy ground and noticed the location the car last made contact with the ground; it was over 200 feet from where the car landed on its side. My mind processed this mechanism of energy. A car travelling at that speed then suddenly coming to a stop even though it slowed slightly from the ground contact was a lot of kinetic energy. There was a very high probability of our patient having internal injuries (internal bleeding) from organ tearing.

I stopped at the police car that was just parked behind the Ambulance. The officer was sitting inside with his door open. I said to the officer: "One of the firefighters told me that the driver was clocked at 239kph. Is that true?"

The police officer replied: "Yes, I clocked him at 239kph before he left the road." I said: "OK, that changes a few things on my end, thanks."

I returned to the Ambulance, opened the back doors and said to my partner: "OK, we have to do a full spinal. I just found out he was clocked by police at 239kmph before he left the off-ramp."

My partner looked surprised and said: "Absolutely...let's do it."

I moved to the Ambulance's outer compartment, removed the clam shell and hard collar kit, and brought it inside. With the help of a fire-fighter, we got the patient onto the clam and strapped him in. It was challenging, as clam shells do not go on very well on soft surfaces like mattresses because the clips at either end have to line up level. After the patient was secured, I began to set up an IV. I straightened his arm and he had large veins, so I choose to go to the AC (Antecubital) at the bend of his arm. I selected a 16G catheter, which could give large volumes of fluid in case his blood pressure dropped. As I was about insert the catheter, I looked back and a semi-trailer was moving past the rear of our Ambulance, only inches from the vehicle. I could not believe it! Could the truck be any closer?

I called out to the Fire Captain to stop the next truck — that happened to be an A-trail tractor trailer unit — until we departed the scene. I finished inserting the IV and the patient barley winced.; he appeared rather sleepy, closing his eyes. I was not concerned initially, as after a major MVI patients get that way as the adrenaline begins to wear off.

After the rear doors were closed and secure, I called out to my partner who was now in the driver's seat: "Smooth Code 3 to S please."

He replied: "Sure, will do. Did you want the cell?"

I said: "Yes, thanks for reminding me."

I reached forward and grabbed the cell phone. We began our transport to the trauma centre. The siren wailed as we went. I grabbed the cell looked up the number for the trauma centre and hit the speed dial.

The trauma nurse answered: "Emerg."

I said: "Hi this is Luciano with BC Ambulance. I am coming in Code 3 with a thirty-five-year-old male patient who was involved in a high speed rollover clocked at 239kph by police. He was found walking on scene. Vitals are currently stable — BP 145/65 Pulse 89 and regular, Respirations 20 and easy. There appears to be no loss of consciousness. He is complaining of mid back pain and right quadrant abdominal pain. C-spine precautions are in place."

The nurse replied: "Did you say he was travelling at 239kph?"

I said: "Yes, clocked by the police."

Nurse replied: "OK, we will make a spot for you."

I said: "OK thanks. We are twelve minutes ETA."

I hung up the phone and continued with documenting my assessment and getting the patient's personal details on the form. If we don't have at least the full name and date-of-birth, the patient cannot be registered. With patients who do not have ID and are found unconscious, they are registered as 'John Doe' until the identity can be confirmed. Lab techs and x-ray techs will not perform tests until there is a wrist band on the patient.

We pulled up to the hospital and backed into a spot. Another crew was at the ER ambulance entrance and as soon as we stopped one of them opened the back doors, peered inside, and said: "You need any help unloading?"

I replied: "Sure, that would be great." Just then, my partner arrived at the back to unload the patient.

We unloaded and wheeled him into the ER reception area. One of the nurses working in the area said: "Is this the guy who was travelling at 239kph?"

I replied: "Yes."

She said: "OK, we are just moving out a patient. As soon as it is clear, you can move him into Trauma 3."

I replied: "OK, I am just going to drop my form of at Admitting and be right back." I walked to another area, dropped off my form at registration, and came back. My partner stayed with the patient. Sometimes patients vomit and being strapped in a clamshell spinal device and unable to protect and clear your airway is not only disconcerting for the patient, but very dangerous for possible aspiration.

A nurse approached us and said: "OK, Trauma 3 is ready for you."

We wheeled the patient into the trauma bay, and relocated the hospital's trauma stretcher already fitted with a slider due to his c-spine precautions. An RT and two nurses arrived a few moments later as we began to unstrap the patient.

On noticing the IV in the patient's left arm the nurse asked: "What size IV did you get there?"

I replied: "A 16."

The nurse looked up with a smile on her face and replied: "Nice."

I said: "Go big or go home" with a chuckle.

Continuing, I said: "Am I giving report now or waiting for the doctor?" Just as I finished the sentence, the ER doctor walked in and made eye contact, a typical non-verbal sign to give my report. Often times there are a lot of non-verbal actions done during trauma transfers; everyone has done this a multitude of times and we all have a role to play in the process.

I began giving my report: "So this is Tylor. He is thirty-four. He was the driver and sole occupant of a car that was clocked at travelling at 239kph when it left an off-ramp of Highway Number One. It travelled through the air approximately two-hundred feet, cleared a concrete barrier, and came to rest on its passenger side in a ditch. All airbags were deployed, and the patient was wearing his seat belt. (The mechanism of the accident is critical in order for the ER doctor to formulate the potential for injuries, also called the 'mechanism of injury'). Tylor self-extricated himself from the car prior to our arrival and was found walking on scene. He says he did not lose consciousness and is complaining of mid to lower back pain, and right upper quadrant abdominal pain. C-spine precautions were put into place as a precautionary measure."

The ER doctor nodded and began his assessment, asking many clarifying questions and requesting orders for tests etc.

I finished off my paperwork for the patient's file and left the trauma room.

The Wallet

We responded to a call to a residence with an elderly patient. My partner was precepting a student paramedic. When we arrived, we were let into a well-kept home. The student did his assessment and we loaded the elderly man, who was experiencing shortness of breath, onto our cot.

The man became anxious once we were ready to depart the residence. The patient said to his wife: "I need my wallet. Where is my wallet?"

The patient's wife replied: "It's safer if you don't bring your wallet to the hospital."

He replied: "Well maybe not, but it's certainly not safer in your purse!!"

I think my partner, the student, and I began laughing and smiling at the same time. That was the funniest thing I had heard all week. The patient maintained a concerned look on his face.

I said: "Sir, how long have you two been married?

The wife answered at the same time he did: "27 years."

I replied: "Priceless....ha ha.! Well, maybe you have this all figured out then."

We wheeled him out to the Ambulance, and the wife held onto his wallet.

'Skunked'

I was working in the metropolitan area of Vancouver on my first night shift. My regular partner for the block had called in sick and my partner for the evening was on holiday recall. It was my drive night, so she would be attending this evening.

We began checking the car for equipment, wiping down the critical areas (front of cab, steering wheel, seat, microphone, radio buttons, clipboard etc,) to prevent cross contamination from the other crew. We always wear gloves during a call, but the cab is where we take them off, drink our beverages and eat, so we want it to be as clean and sanitary as possible. The wipes we use literally kill anything on contact.

It was now 0130hrs and I badly needed some caffeine. My normal solution go to was Starbucks, as I liked the stronger flavour of their coffee. But, at this time of the evening, there were none open, so that left Tim Hortons and McDonald's. It was always a toss-up for me, as the newer dark roast at Tim's was almost acceptable and the food choices were better if I decided to grab a snack.

We pulled up to the Tim's and, just then, the CAD sounded: "Blip...blip...blip." My partner, Janet, looked at the screen as I said: "If that is routine, I am going in to grab my coffee"

Janet replied: "It's a pre-alert."

I waited a few more seconds and the CAD again sounded: "Blip...blip."

Janet said: "It's wait for the 5s...grab your coffee."

Halfway out the door, I said: "Do you want anything?"

Janet replied: "No, I'm good thanks."

I grabbed my coffee and a BLT as it was not busy and they prepared it quickly. I did not want to delay heading to this call even though it was a wait. I climbed back into the car, opened my sandwich, took a few bites then headed toward the call. The streets were quiet at this time of early morning and the call was only about eight minutes away.

As I drove, Janet said: "This is a wait due to violent history with first responders. Police have been requested. He was apparently assaulted earlier in the evening."

I pulled up a few blocks away and turned the car off, leaving the park light on along with the much-needed music radio.

I spun the CAD toward me and read the dispatch notes. Just then the CAD sounded again: "Blip...blip." It read:

- Police not attending as they attended earlier today for the same incident
- Dispatch requests police, crew will not enter without police on scene due to history of violence of patient
- Police will attend

"Great!" I said. "The police did not want to attend at first...apparently dealt with this guy before."

Janet replied: "Well it will probably be a while. This won't be a priority call then."

We both chilled, with the radio in the background, playing 80s music and top 40. I was just about to watch some Netflix when the CAD sounded: "Blip...blip."

I looked at the CAD and it read: "SAFE Police on scene."

I drove up to a police car sitting across from the residence of the narrow Vancouver Street. The officer got out and approached my window.

I said: "So what's up with this guy? Sounds like you have a history with him from the notes on our CAD." The officer replied: "Well, let's put it this way: I have personally attended to his residence at least twenty times. He is a drain on our resources and the system. He calls so often our supervisors will screen the call and decide if we are going to attend."

I said: "Oh, OK. Geez, well from the notes he has been aggressive to first responders so that is why we insisted on you attending."

The officer replied: "Well, this guy is in a wheelchair. His mother lives upstairs.; she is old and frail. He is more bark than bite...not really capable of doing much."

I laughed out loud then said: "Seriously! In a wheelchair? So basically take a step back and you are safe. Wow. OK, well let's find out what is going on tonight." I looked over at Janet and she just rolled her eyes and sighed.

We got out and walked over to the house. Despite what we knew about the patient, Janet did grab the kit from the side-access door of the car. We entered a walkway and the cop new that the two-story residence had a rented unit to the right, while the patient lived to the left when facing the house.

We looked through the blinds and noticed the man lying on his bed. I could see he was breathing. He did not respond to our calls through the slightly open window, calls back by our dispatcher, or knocks on his window. We discussed forced entry and could not decide, as he was obviously breathing with no obvious injury. The cop called his supervisor to attend. After the cop went around the back and found a patio door unlocked, he came back to get us. We walked in with the cop in the lead. As we entered his living room, the TV was on. We called out to the patient; his name was Jerry.

I said: "Jerry, Jerry, it's the Paramedics and police."

Jerry groaned, "Huh," and moved his head a bit.

I said again: "Jerry, why did you call 911? Why are we here?"

Jerry again groaned: "Huh...I was assaulted."

I looked at Janet and asked: "Do you want to question him?"

Janet replied: "No, you are doing fine. Go ahead."

I grabbed the kit, placed the Spo2 probe on one of his fingers, and checked his radial pulse. His pulse was regular and easily felt. The Spo2 read 95% and had a rate of 79bpm.

I said: "Jerry, are you hurt anyplace?"

Jerry replied in a moan again: "Yes, here." He motioned to the centre of his chest.

I asked Janet what meds he was on. She observed a blister pack and a few other random bottles nearby. The cop said: "He is known to use street drugs and prescription meds."

I said: "Janet, I'll just grab the cot as you complete your assessment, as we are obviously going to have to take this guy in. His LOC is decreased."

Janet replied: "Yes, looks like we are."

As I walked out, I began thinking of moving him onto our cot. He was obese, missing a leg, and with decreased LOC probably not a lot of help. Prior to exiting the house I flipped on the outside light and proceeded down the walkway from the house toward the sidewalk. Just before I passed by a low, three foot high brick wall, I noticed an animal. It was black and white, very furry, and scurried around the wall into the plant garden. I immediately identified it as a skunk and thought 'Oh what a cute little skunk.' I was tired, as it was now 0230, and was not thinking very clearly even with the coffee and BLT. I continued walking without a pause. As I approached the rear of the vehicle I thought: 'Wow is that ever lucky that that skunk did not spray me — that was close.'

Just then it hit me...the strongest most acrid smell I had ever smelled before – it was skunk. It took my breath away for a few moments. I had never smelled a skunk that strong before in my life. At first, I thought, 'Oh the skunk sprayed after I walked by.' I paused a moment and shone my flashlight on my pants to see if I could see anything on them, such as droplets; it looked like there was. I put my foot on the back bumper and smelled my pant leg...it was strong. I thought 'I must have been sprayed.'

The smell in my nose was actually dissipating somewhat now, so I was not having the feeling that I could not breath like before.

I decided to head back into the call to confirm it was on my person before I put us out of service and called a second unit to attend to transport the patient. I walked back inside, motioned for my partner to come toward me, and she approached. I said: "I think I was sprayed by a skunk. Can you smell anything on me?" There was a momentary pause. Then, all of a sudden, she got this awful look on her face and began backing away."

She replied: "Yes, you were sprayed by a skunk!...Ahhh its awful!"

With that, I turned and walked back to the Ambulance and called Dispatch on the radio: "98A2."

Dispatch: "98A2."

"98A2. We are out of service. Will require a second care routine. I will give you a landline with details."

Dispatch: "98A2 10-4. You will have 89A from quarters."

"10-4."

I made a cell call to Dispatch and explained the situation, then called one of our road supervisors and also explained what happened. I then looked up 'how to decontaminate skunk.' My Internet search revealed that a mixture of hydrogen peroxide and baking soda would work. I then called the local hospital and spoke to the triage nurse about getting a bottle of hydrogen peroxide to decontaminate myself. She told me they had some.

My partner appeared from the house with the two police officers a few moments later. After some discussions held at a distance from me, it was decided that I had, in fact, been sprayed by the skunk. Fortunately, by this time I could barely smell the skunk on me. My suspicion was that the body's olfactory nerves (sense of smell) shut down the odor to protect the senses. The other crew arrived and, after a lot of laughing (well, it was funny even though I was looking forward to cleaning up), they grabbed me a Tyvek suit (white overalls, worn typically to protect us from bio-hazard) to change into and bagged my contaminated uniform. I climbed in the back, stripped down to my underwear.

Using Sea Cleanse, I sprayed my thighs with the antibacterial soap. Unfortunately, it did not remove the acrid stench. After bagging my clothing, I reappeared wearing the Tyvek suit and black boots; there was more laughter. We departed shortly afterwards. I told my partner, Janet, that I would sit in the back. She closed the Plexiglas window shortly after pulling out; apparently the smell was leaching out of the double plastic bags I had put my clothing into.

We arrived at the hospital shortly and, after exiting, I headed straight for the dumpster and deposited my bag of contaminated clothing. My road supervisor suggested I have it dry cleaned. Well, I certainly was not transporting that in my car and no drycleaner was going to want to even think about cleaning that! It was disposed of permanently. Another crew member appeared from the ER doors shortly afterwards with a small bottle of hydrogen peroxide.

He said: "I was handed this by the triage nurse. She said you would be here shortly."

I replied: "Thanks."

Janet had gone inside to get me a set of hospital scrubs to change into and the triage nurse told her that her clothing had also been contaminated with skunk and to leave the ER area. Since we did not have baking soda my partner drove us to a 24-hour Shoppers Drug Mart (thankfully they have those!) She bought three large boxes of baking soda and we were on our way!

Once back at the station, I initially mopped and wiped the inside of the car down then I made the magic potion in a bucket and headed for the shower. After scrubbing my skin below the neck with the solution (I didn't want my hair to be peroxide white after this event!) I used soap and again scrubbed myself down with soap and shampoo. I changed into the scrubs and was told I did not smell of skunk anymore (Eureka!)

I headed home shortly afterward, as it was now 4:30 in the morning... what a night!

Helicopter Crash

We were sitting at our station in a smaller town when my partner walked up to me and said: "There is a possible helicopter crash that happened about twenty minutes from here. We may be getting a call."

I replied: "Oh, really, how did you hear that?"

He said: "I have a fire pager and I have been monitoring a call that just came in." Just then, the pagers sounded: "Beep...beep...beep.... shhhhhhh.... 43A1...Code 3 call...43A Code 3 call."

My partner was in the bay, so I headed outside, jumped in the Ambulance on the attendant's side, and looked at the CAD.

- Event: Aircraft Crash
- Persons involved: Unknown injuries, unknown number of persons, unknown nature of injuries.
- Location: Rural area, near a dyke
- Units: 43A1, 480 (medi-vac helicopter)
- PD: Units responding
- FD: Fire Department responding
- Notes:
  - 1400- Location of crash site to be determined
  - 1401- Significant event supervisors paged
  - 1402- Possible helicopter
  - 1403- May have crashed in the water

My partner got in and I said: "Looks like you were right. We got the call to the helicopter crash." He and I and pulled out of the bay, activated the lights and siren, and headed toward the scene.

Dispatch: "43A be advised 480 is on standby. Please advise when you get on scene if they are required."

My partner grabbed the mike and said: "43A – 10-4."

As we proceeded to the call I said: "The CAD does not say anything about JRCC being notified. I wonder if they called them."

My partner was concentrating on driving and just nodded as he adjusted the siren tones to alert the heavy traffic. My partner was pushing it to get to the call as we were a long way away and the only unit assigned at this time due to limited resources. 480 was the only other unit on standby and that was a helicopter for medivac if we needed it.

I picked up the cell phone and speed-dialed our channel operator. Each radio channel has its own dispatcher.

The operator answered: "Channel 3."

I said: "Hi, it's 43A. Just wanted to know if JRCC has been notified?"

Dispatch: "GR...who?"

I replied: "JRCC."

Getting rather annoyed at this point I replied: "Rescue Centre."

Dispatch: "Oh....umm...not sure. Let me check with the charge."

I replied: "Well, seeing that this is an aircraft crash, they should be notified and put on standby."

Dispatch: "I will check it out"

I replied: "Sure, OK."

I hung up the phone and turned to my partner and said: "Gotta love the new dispatchers. First, does not even know what 'JRCC' stands for. Then, when I say 'rescue centre,' he pauses, thinking about it...you would think that it would be on their call out list."

My partner glanced over: "Yeah, well this should not surprise us — seems to be common lately."

We continued on, my partner weaving through traffic as we left the city limits and entered farming areas. As we approached the crash site that had yet to be found, the CAD sounded: "Blip...blip."

I read the CAD: "Rescue Centre notified."

'Great,' I thought, 'we are fifteen minutes into this call and they only notified JRCC after I asked them.'

Our CAD mapping system was not working properly, so I was trying to keep up on our location, so we would not pass the road we were to turn onto, as I knew we were getting close. Problem was, every time

I would zoom in on the CAD map, it would jump to where our vehicle was on the map with every update. Often the updates would be heard but nothing obvious would be noticed on the screen. The system was not set up to highlight or otherwise indicate new changes; yet another fail with the CAD system. There were about ten things that could have changed to make the system work better.

After a few more non-noticed updates on the CAD, I pushed the mapping button to see where the road was to turn onto. I said: "So we are supposed to turn right onto Oxford Road." I looked up from the CAD and noticed Oxford Rd whiz past us as we raced toward the call.

Continuing, I said: "That was Oxford Rd we just passed. Sorry, man. We can take the next turn and loop in toward the call that way also."

My partner, clearly a bit annoyed that I missed the turn, said: "I'll just spin around and go back, I don't want to go any farther out of the way than we have to."

I was silent as he turned the Ambulance around on the two-lane highway. He zoomed back to the turn and headed toward the last location the Code 6 (fire department) gave for the crash site. We noticed a fire truck up ahead and proceeded toward it even though the road we were supposed to turn onto was at road junction we had just reached.

My partner said: "Well, no point in going to the left when the fire truck is to the right and up ahead. Clearly they have not updated the location of the crash site."

The CAD had been blipping as we drove with updates, including notifying our regional and local supervisors who were also responding to the crash site. Everyone wanted to be part of the action on this call. We don't get very many helicopter crashes and it was exciting for everyone to be involved. After we arrived at the fire truck in the intersection, we were directed toward a dike road up ahead. My partner was familiar with the area and it led us to a narrow single-lane road with drop-offs on each side sloping down toward the farm fields twenty feet below the slope. The road was a bit rough, but not as bad as expected, and my partner maintained speeds of 50kph as we closed in on the crash site.

When we finally arrived, there was a string of vehicles along the roadway leading to the exact location of the crash site.

Dispatch: "43A."

My partner grabbed the mike: "43A."

Dispatch: "Let me know what resources you need."

My partner replied slightly sarcastically: "Sure, as soon as we get to the crash site we will let you know."

We exited the Ambulance and were met by a couple of firefighters. The Captain said: "The pilot is conscious and walked away from the crash site. My guys have c-spine in place. You guys want us to bring your stretcher down?"

I replied: "Well, I wanted to assess the situation first."

I grabbed my kit, a hard collar, and the O2. My partner and I began picking our way along the roadway to the crash site. There were four police cars and a fire rescue truck before we reached a full-sized pickup truck with a man sitting on the tailgate surrounded by firefighters. I looked to the right and in the field below the slope of the dyke I could see the wreckage of the helicopter. From my vantage point, it looked pretty bad, only resembling a heap of scrap metal.

As I approached, one of the firefighters turned to me and said: "This is Sanjo. He is the pilot. He walked away from the crash site. He has a pretty serious head injury. We have c-spine in place." I responded: "OK guys, let me get in there and take a look please." The firefighters not holding c-spine or holding a large trauma dressing to his head moved aside.

I looked at the man. He was in his early thirties, was conscious, made eye contact, and was sitting upright on his own. There was obvious blood on his shirt but no deformity to any of his body limbs.

I said: "Hi, my name is Luke, I am a Paramedic. I am going to ask you some questions. Keep your head still and do not move your head or neck, OK?"

The pilot replied: "OK, I'm OK."

I said: "I just need to check you out and see if you have any injuries."

The pilot replied: "I'm OK."

I began my assessment with his head. I briefly removed the trauma dressing the firefighters had over the wound; it was a two-centimetre laceration to the scalp that had been bleeding. I re-covered the wound with the firefighter holding pressure. I examined his neck, but he did not feel pain or discomfort. I exposed his chest, and he had a few abrasions, but no punctures or obvious bruising or trauma. Using my stethoscope, I auscultated his chest anterior and posterior for equal air entry and any pain.

I asked him if he had lost consciousness and what other aches and pains he had. He mentioned a few things — his shoulder, head, and leg — but he was obviously in emotional shock from the crash and adrenaline was still pumping through his body. The bad part of adrenaline is that it protects the body from feeling pain and therefore masks injuries until it wears off. This is important to know so precautions can be taken to protect the patient by observing the mechanism of the crash to determine possible forces that may cause injuries that would otherwise not be noticed. That is why in trauma patients it is especially important to do hands-on exams; otherwise, injuries are often missed.

My partner returned from the crash site and said: "What do you want to do? Do you need anything?"

I replied: "Yes, I am going to do a full spinal, so we will need the clam and stretcher." The Fire Captain standing beside him said: "We can grab that for you." My partner said: "OK sure. I will come back to the car with you."

He turned to me as he approached: "Do you need the kit anymore?"

I replied: "Yes, just want to dress and bandage the head wound then you can take it back." I pulled out some dressings and roller gauze, and wrapped the head wound, relieving the firefighter from holding pressure.

A C-collar was applied around his neck and I instructed the pilot to not move his head.

When the remainder of the equipment arrived, I asked the pilot to stand. When he did so, he said that he felt slightly light-headed. He took the two steps to the clamshell (split backboard device used to secure and stabilize spinal precaution patients). He was assisted to the supine position, strapped in, and four of us wheeled him along the gravel dyke road toward the Ambulance parked approximately 500 feet away.

After loading him in, my partner said: "Do you need to do anything before we leave?"

I replied: "Yes, I want to get a line in him just in case he has any internal injuries. His veins are up right now, so it won't delay transport."

He said: "OK, just let me know when you want to get going?"

I replied: "OK, sounds good."

I prepared my IV supplies, including a 1000cc bag of normal saline, put on the tourniquet, and began looking for veins in his arm. Only the patient and myself were in the back of the Ambulance that was running with the air conditioning buzzing in the background. I said: "Sanjo, I'm going to start an IV and then we are going to head to the hospital to get you assessed by an emergency room doctor. Want to make sure you don't have any injuries that are not apparent right now."

Sanjo replied: "Sure...OK. I guess I am not going to fly again. I destroyed that helicopter."

I said: "Sure you will...what do you think insurance is for?"

Sanjo replied: "You think? I don't think so. I think they won't let me fly anymore after that."

I continued with my IV start. I decided that I wanted to go with a large-bore IV, so found a garden hose vein at his left AC, grabbed a 16G catheter (it looks like a pipe it's so big), and, after telling Sanjo he would feel a poke, jabbed it in. It went in perfectly. I connected the IV tubing and let if flow; it was such a large catheter that it streamed down the drip chamber so fast it was a steady stream rather than drips. After securing the line and taping it up I rechecked all the straps on the clam, placed quick release straps on the patient's head and foot end on my side of the clam, connecting it to the main cot so he could be flipped sideways. (This would also keep him strapped in the spinal position in case he vomited suddenly en route to the hospital, a good possibility with head injuries). I re-checked the dressing on his head and it was soaking through. I checked the firmness of the dressing, but surmised that it was due to the change of position from sitting to lying down.

I put another abdominal dressing over the one already there and, using some bulk padding, wedged it in between the clam and his head to apply pressure without having me hold it during transport.

My partner was waiting in the driver's seat, engine running. I went forward and poked my head through the opening. "Can you hand me the phone, and we can head out anytime, Code 3, due to mechanism and distance from hospital."

He replied: "Sure I will light it up when we get on the main road."

I said: "Sounds good to me! Thanks."

Because there was no place to turn around my partner had to back up along the single lane dyke road with sloped sides on either side until we made it to an intersection about half a kilometre from where the incident was. Once we were on paved roads, he activated the emergency equipment (lights and sirens) and drove smoothly but quickly toward the nearest appropriate hospital. This hospital had a heli-pad adjacent to it. I chose this hospital in case my patient's condition deteriorated; in that eventuality, I would activate a medi-vac helo to meet us at the hospital and bypass the ER.

I called the hospital once we were on the hard-surface roads. The Triage nurse answered: "Triage."

I said: "Hi, this BCAS calling. I'm en route, Code 3, with an adult male patient who was the pilot in a helicopter crash. He walked from the scene. His vitals are stable at this time; BP 160/90 Pulse 86, Resp 20. He has an open head laceration approximately three centimetres that is controlled, with no loss of consciousness. C-spine precautions are in place due to mechanism, and I have an IV running. Our ETA is fourteen minutes.

The triage nurse replied: "Did you say he is a helicopter pilot?"

I replied: "Yes, and you are the most appropriate hospital based on his condition."

The triage nurse replied: "OK, because you would normally go to a trauma centre, right?"

I said: "Yes, if his condition and injuries warranted it I would, but he does not fit the criteria at this time."

The triage nurse replied: "OK, we will be ready for you."

I said: "Great, see you soon."

While en route to the hospital I talked with the patient and monitored his vital signs — especially his BP and LOC — looking for changes that might warrant a higher priority CTAS[6] level.

We arrived at the hospital in a short time, unloaded the stretcher, and wheeled him through the ER doors. The ER was very busy with overflow stretchers lined up along the walls of the ward. We stopped long enough to hand the pink copy to admitting. The Triage nurse said: "Is this the helicopter pilot?" As she said this, a few paramedics standing nearby with their patients turned and looked toward us. It is unusual for crews to bring in helicopter crash patients — let's just say it does not happen often.

The triage nurse said: "OK take him directly to Trauma 1."

"OK."

We wheeled him toward the trauma room, past all the carts cluttered in the hallway. There were staff, visitors and patients everywhere. One thing about when we call ahead with a trauma patient: we move right to the front of the line!

As we passed an ER a doctor said, "Is that the helicopter pilot?"

I replied: "Yes"

The ER doctor just looked at me with this look of 'Why did you bring him here?'

We entered the trauma room, moved and adjusted the trauma stretcher and moved our cot beside to transfer our patient over to the hospital one. Just then, an ER nurse arrived with some paperwork. We lifted the clam onto the hospital stretcher and removed it, leaving the hard collar in place, and hung the IV line. Within a few moments, the trauma room had three other staff: another nurse, a lab tech, and an x-ray tech; they were joined shortly by the ER doctor we passed in the hallway.

As soon as the doctor entered I looked at him and began my report: "This is Sanjo. He is a thirty-five-year-old who was the pilot and sole

---

6   Canadian Triage Acuity Scale

occupant in a helicopter crash. The helicopter crashed from a hover height of approximately twenty feet and drifted sideways off a dyke down a slope and collided with a grass field. Sanjo did not lose consciousness, self-extricated himself prior to arrival, and walked from the scene. On arrival we found him sitting on the back tailgate of a pick-up truck. C-spine was in place with the fire department. He was alert, orientated. He has a three-centimetre laceration on the top his head that is controlled. He is also complaining of right shoulder pain, but is able to ambulate his arm, with decreased range or motion, and no peripheral paralysis or numbness. He is also complaining of some left thigh pain but is able to weight bear and walked a few steps to the cot. His last vitals were 160/78 pulse 78, resp 20, and easy sats 98%. C-spine precautions have been put in place due to mechanism and a 16G IV was started in his left AC."

There was concurrent activity as I gave my report: nurses were stripping his clothing, lab techs taking blood, and the x-ray tech was nearby with the portable x-ray machine.

The doctor said, "OK, thanks," still looking at with me with that 'Why did you bring him here?' look.

He began his assessment asked the patient a number of questions as he did. He explained what they were going to do as far as tests to rule out any serious injury. After the doctor completed his exam and issued orders to the staff, he looked over at me with a look of 'OK, I see why you brought him here other than a trauma centre'; I nodded as if I understood the 'look' he gave me.

My partner had already left the trauma room with our equipment and I stood nearby and finished my paperwork. By the time I got back to the car, my partner had put everything back, re-stocked as necessary, mopped out the back of the car, and was sitting in the driver's seat waiting for me.

We pulled away from the hospital and talked about the call briefly as we headed back toward our home area.

Bike on sidewalk

The day crew had just got back to the station when the hotline rang! My partner picked up the phone and said: "Station 34....yes, OK but we will need a few minutes to check the car." She hung up and said to me: "We have a pre-alert on the CAD." I replied: "OK, guess it's time to go. Surprise! We have a call waiting...ha ha!"

My partner said: "Yeah, no kidding. Nothing ever changes."

We headed downstairs, went outside to our awaiting Ambulance, and began doing the essential checks: Oxygen, jump kit, spinal kit, suction, AED. My partner was the attendant tonight, so I started the car, checked the emergency lights, and logged into the CAD. Once I logged on, the CAD sounded: "Blip...blip...blip." My partner said: "We have a pedestrian struck, about four minutes from here."

The CAD read:
- Location: Main Road and Spike Street
- Response: Code 3
- Type: Pedestrian struck
- Call source: Person on scene
- Units: 34A
- Remarks: Cyclist struck, near Night and Day restaurant, Status: Unknown, Injuries: Unknown, Sex: Unknown, Age: Unknown

I replied: "OK we will be right there." She finished checking the equipment and climbed in on the right (attendant seat).

As we screamed down the road toward the call, the traffic was heavy, and people were (of course) doing stupid things to impede our progress toward the scene, such as blocking us by stopping directly in front of us even though there was a clear lane beside us.

We pulled up to the scene to see a man standing on the sidewalk near the Night and Day restaurant. There was a small two-door red car nearby and another man nearby. We also noticed a bike leaning against a lamp pole. After stopping I said: "Oh this should be good! Glad we drove Code 3 for this!"

My partner replied: "Yeah no kidding. This looks real serious." I could hear the sarcasm in her voice very clearly.

We both got out and headed toward the man standing near the bike, who was talking on his cell phone. He was still talking after we were standing three feet from him. He had some obvious abrasions on his right shoulder and right elbow, and there was a bit of blood oozing from the wounds. Other than that, he was moving around in such an erratic manner that nothing else seemed wrong with him.

I said to him: "Sir, we need you to hang up the phone, so my partner can ask you some questions and check you out."

The patient continued to talk on his cell phone, then finally hung up.

The patient said: "Are the cops coming? That guy hit me, knocked me off my bike. I can't believe it! I want the cops to come and give him a ticket. I can't believe this...look at my bike!" As he spoke, he waved his arms around in an erratic manner.

My partner approached him and began questioning him about the accident (did he hit his head, have neck pain, lose consciousness etc.) As she questioned him, I walked over to the other man standing near his car. I looked at the car and there was no noticeable damage to it. The man had a very reluctant sheepish detached look on his face...more of a stunned look.

I said: "Hi, my name is Luke. Can you tell me what happened?"

The man replied in an East Indian accent: "Yes, I was exiting the parking lot and all of a sudden this man appeared on his bike right in front of my car. He was going so fast and I could not stop, so I smashed into him. And now he has been yelling at me." Before I could say anything, the patient came over and started yelling at the driver again.

"I can't believe you fucking hit me. Geeeez, just look at my arm." (He motioned to the road rash on his shoulder.) "Why don't you look where you are going? You can't just come out, you are supposed to look...

Look at my bike, I can't even peddle it." The driver did not reply after this verbal expulsion.

I said to the patient: "Sir, I need you to get back over there, away from this man. The police are on the way and will sort out fault."

The patient replied: "Fault?...It's clearly his fault, he hit me! Knocked me down!"

My partner said: "Let's go back over there and let me finish checking you out, OK?"

The patient replied: "Yeah OK, but when are the police get here, I want him charged."

The patient and my partner moved away from the driver. I called on my portable radio, asking for an ETA of the police; the dispatcher advised they would be there shortly.

When the police arrived in an unmarked police car, the patient again began his erratic behavior — shouting, moving his arms, and waving all about. My partner came up to me a few minutes after they arrived, after of the officers began to interview the patient. She said: "That guy smells like mouthwash, and he is chewing gum. I think he is impaired with something." I replied: "You should make sure the police know." She said: "Yes, I will."

I walked over to one of the police officers and we discussed the incident. The officer made it very clear that the patient was in the wrong for not wearing a helmet and riding on the sidewalk, and it would be clearly written in the report to ICBC. After some further discussion with the patient about if he actually wanted to be checked out by a doctor, he decided to come with us. We placed his bike in the back of the Ambulance and secured it with a short strap. When we arrived at the hospital, my partner gave report to triage, and the patient was directed to the waiting room.

When we departed the hospital, my partner and I discussed the call. "What a piece of work he was," she said.

I replied: "Yeah, no kidding, what an idiot. The cops told me that they could have written him two tickets and they were going to make it very clear in their ICBC report that he was on the sidewalk and not wearing a helmet."

She said: "If he was not riding like that, he would not have been hit in the first place." We drove alone in silence for a moment when the CAD suddenly sounded: "Blip...blip...blip." Another call.

Stabbed in the Chest

It was a normal non-stop day in the metropolitan Vancouver area. My regular partner was on vacation, so someone was in on OT. She and I were just pulling into our station, looking forward to perhaps putting our feet up for even thirty minutes, when that dreaded sound was heard: "Blip...blip...blip." Another call!!

My partner groaned: "Really...again!" She spun the CAD toward her and said: "We have a stabbing!"

I replied: "Really?" suddenly feeling my adrenaline kick in. We Paramedics are a strange bunch; the worse the call, the more we want to go to it. Perhaps it's the rush of the unknown, or, if we can keep the person alive, the challenge of our abilities and limits.

My partner said, "OK, head to," and gave me the general direction of the call. "I will put it in the GPS and guide you in."

I replied: "OK, I'll light it up." I activated the emergency lights, turned on the siren, and checked for traffic stopping (as, often, people just drive past, staring at us with all our emergency equipment activated). I spun the Amb around and punched it (pushed on the accelerator to the floor). The engine roared as it picked up speed. This was a real call, and could be life-threatening, so time was of essence, but we still a had to make it there safe and not get into a crash on the way.

The CAD blipped as I drove, making almost full-stops at red lights, and going into oncoming traffic often as there was a lot of traffic on this four-lane city roadway. As we approached yet another intersection that was blocked by a red light, I went into the oncoming lane, alternating the siren as I went. Near the intersection, I noticed a police car with its emergency equipment activated, moving in the direction I was planning on heading. I immediately assumed the car was going to the stabbing as, with high priority calls, everyone wants to be a part of the action. As I approached the intersection and turned in the direction of the police car, I noticed it slowed to almost a stop. I immediately presumed the officer noticed we were heading to the call so was going to run the call together. (It's safer to have two emergency vehicles travel close together through traffic and intersections, rather than a distance apart, as traffic will continue to drive as the first one passes by). The cop was driving fast (as they normally do) and I pushed it as we weaved through traffic and intersections.

We arrived at the call and there were a number of police vehicles and officers walking about. I opened the window and shouted out to one of them: "Where is the patient?"

The officer nearest to us pointed to the location and said: "Just ahead in the doorway."

I replied, "OK thanks," and drove ahead to where we could see the commotion of people in an open doorway leading to a commercial business. There was a female police officer holding something on top of a man lying in the doorway.

I said to my partner: "I'll grab the O2 and cot and meet you at the doorway." She replied, "OK sounds good," excited the Ambulance, and grabbed the jump kit from the side compartment as I headed back to get the O2 secured to the back door. I pulled out the cot, let the carriage drop to the ground and threw the O2 bottle on top, and wheeled it to the curb. I grabbed the O2 and headed over to assist my partner who was already assessing the patient. The patient was a young Caucasian male in his early 20s; he was conscious, talking, and did not appear to be in any respiratory distress. A female police officer was holding a large blood-soaked towel on top of his chest.

I said to my partner: "What do you need? Do you need a chest seal?" (An Asherman Chest Seal is a round, disk-like adhesive bandage that has a short rubber tube sticking out and is designed to adhere to the chest and allow air to escape if there is an open pneumothorax, but will prevent air from entering by way of a one-way flutter valve).

My partner replied: "I have one, but not sure if there is penetration to the chest cavity."

I said: "Well, let's take the towel off and cut off the shirt and get a better look."

She replied: "OK."

The officer removed the blood-soaked towel and my partner pulled the bloody shirt away to reveal a very large slashing laceration across the right side of his upper chest, approximately 15cm long, and a second laceration on the left side of his chest approximately 8cm long. There was blood oozing from the wounds but no apparent escaping air. I grabbed a large trauma dressing from the kit, tore it from its packaging, and placed it over the chest, covering both wounds.

Just then, we heard a female's voice behind us: "Don't worry about that, just get him out of there." It was a familiar sound of an ALS Paramedic. Neither my partner nor I replied, and we continued to treat the patient. I pulled out my scissors and the ALS paramedic said: "Cut off his shirt and get him on the cot".

I was getting annoyed now; my inside voice was thinking: 'Why doesn't she just let us do our job, and maybe actually ask what she and her partner can do for us rather than barking orders at us. She does not even know what we have.' After ruling out C-Spine injuries we sat the man up and I cut the shirt off to fully expose the rest of the man's chest and back. There were no exit wounds or other wounds to the back of his chest. We did notice anther laceration to his right shoulder at the deltoid muscle, approximately 5cm long. We stood him up.

The ALS Paramedic said: "Get him over on the cot. Don't worry about doing anything else."

By now, my inside voice was fuming, and I think I actually bit my tongue in order to prevent myself from saying anything to her. I was thinking, 'Does she not realize that we know what we are doing and don't need to be treated like untrained bystanders?' The man stood, up and walked the few steps over to the cot where we laid him down. It was apparent that he was clearly in stable condition at this time, considering that he could do that. It was decided that my partner would drive him into the hospital and I would follow in our car.

I cleaned up the remainder of the scene and drove routine to the hospital. When I arrived at the hospital, the patient was in the trauma room surrounded by a team of nurses, technicians and an ER doctor. I stayed and watched for a few minutes, then left the trauma room. After cleaning and stocking our car, we left the scene. Before I left the hospital, I spoke to the female paramedic's partner about her on-scene behavior. He said that it was an ongoing issue and he had to deal with multiple incidents where she acted and said inappropriate things during a call. Apparently, this was a theme for her during calls. I rolled my eyes and walked back to my Ambulance.

The leg waxing

We had just checked our car when the hotline rang. My partner, who was driving, came out and said we had a Code 3 call. The CAD had the call on the screen. I had a student this block, so was attending for four days in a row. I took a look at the CAD after my partner entered the address into the GPS on the dash. It read:|

- Location: Cactus Club
- Alert: Code 3
- Event: Laceration to foot, severe bleed
- Notes: Staff advise, Pt was cut to foot by broken glass

My partner activated the emergency equipment and the siren screamed as we proceeded through moderate traffic to the call. When we were only three minutes from the call, the CAD blipped:

- Alert: Code 2

The dispatcher said: "40A, copy the call has been downgraded to routine." My partner grabbed the mike and said: "10-4."

By this point, we were only a block away. We entered a mall area and parked just outside an open door at the side of the Cactus Club. I said to my student: "OK, we are here. Just grab the kit for now and a few extra telfa and abdominal pads and we will check it out."

He replied: "Yup, I have them right here."

We all exited the Ambulance and headed toward the open side employee door with a well-dressed man standing nearby. As we approached, he greeted us and told us the staff member was inside. We entered the narrow hallway and noticed a number of very attractive young women wearing black dresses and heels. (Cactus club always hired the most attractive women to work in their restaurants — a nice change of environment from our normal calls in back alleys and dirty homes).

We were directed to the back, where a young woman (twenty-six-years-old) wearing a skirt and top was sitting on a chair and a young man was holding a white towel on her ankle. She was alert, conscious, and did not look like she was in any distress. As we approached, she turned and looked at us. I said: "Hi."

She immediately replied: "OK, before you come any closer there is something very important I have to tell you." I paused, as did my student behind me and my partner behind him.

She continued: "I don't want you to look at my legs."

Of course, I immediately looked at her legs, somewhat distracted as they were very nice. She continued, in a very serious manner: "I did not have time to wax my legs. They are hairy, and I don't want you to look at them."

I paused a moment as I took this information in. Here was a gorgeous young woman, dressed very nicely, with a bright, positive smile, telling me to not look at her legs because she did not have time to wax them? I almost didn't know what to say as I once again gazed toward her legs. Not noticing any hair, I was puzzled by her statement.

I replied, "OK, you are joking, right?" and I laughed.

She said: "No, I'm serious. Please don't look at them...I'm so embarrassed."

I approached the staff member holding the white partially blood-soaked towel around her ankle and moved in where I could see the wound.

I said: "My name is Luciano."

She replied: "Mine is Tanya."

I said: "OK, can you tell me what happened?"

She replied: "Well, I was standing by the front entrance, a glass fell from a tray, smashed on the floor, and shards of glass flew into my leg."

I replied: "OK, did you or anyone" — looking over at the other staff member who had been holding the towel on her leg — "else notice any glass left in the wound?" The staff member said: "I didn't see anything before I put the towel on her leg."

She replied: "Me neither. I don't think there is anything."

I removed the towel and the bleeding was now under control. My examination revealed two small lacerations. One was approximately 2cm long and the other 1cm, but they were deep enough and in an area that would require two or three sutures.

I turned to my student and had him hand me dressings as I placed them over the wound and wrapped it in a roller gauze. I said to the patient, Tanya, "OK, let's get you some footwear and take you up to the hospital for some sutures."

Tanya replied: "What, really? I have to go to the hospital?"

I replied: "Yes, you certainly do. You will need a few sutures."

With the help of some of her colleagues, we found some flip-flops rather than the three-inch heels she was wearing, and she walked to the Amb and was seated in the back in the captain's chair.

During the drive to the hospital, we chatted and laughed about the waxing comment. I told Tanya I was writing a book and her story would definitely be in it. Upon arrival at the hospital, Tanya again told the Triage nurse about having not waxed her legs and how embarrassed she was. I was almost laughing out loud; I could not believe it. We escorted her to the minor treatment area, gave the bedside nurse our report, then left.

On a return from another call, we brought another patient to the minor treatment area and decided to check up on Tanya to see if she had her sutures yet. The ER doctor was just setting up a suture tray when my student and I walked over. I said in a sarcastic tone: "What, you have not had your sutures yet?" smiling at the ER doctor. Smiling, the doctor said, "Yes, well I have been busy."

I replied: "Had I known, I could have put those in for you." The doctor, knowing I was a military medic trained in suturing, replied: "Yes, I'm sure you could have. What would you have used"?

I replied: "Uhmmm…probably Xylocaine with 2% epinephrine, and 4-0 Dermalon." The doctor replied: "Oh really…4-0 Dermalon…I am going to use something a bit finer: 4-0 chromo, more often used in plastics. Gives a neater finish." I replied: "Nice, less of a battle scar," as I looked over at Tanya and smiled.

Looking at Tanya, I said: "So, did you tell the Doctor about you not waxing your legs?"

The doctor paused and looked up at me as I said this with a bit of surprise on his face.

Smiling, Tanya replied: "No, I didn't."

I replied: "What? Seriously, you have told everyone else so far…ha ha."

Tanya replied: "Well, guess I didn't think it was important this time."

I said: "Well, we will head back out. I see you are in capable hands," glancing over at the doctor who was now finishing up his second suture. Tanya replied: "Thanks again. Have a great rest of your shift."

We left the treatment area and returned to our car.

Too early to go

We had just got our car from the night shift, and my partner was in the back, checking stock, when I said I wanted to get a coffee at Starbucks before our first call. He decided to stay in the back while I drove.

After about six minutes, the CAD suddenly sounded: "Blip...blip...blip." I said out loud: "I knew we would not make it to grab a coffee." I looked at the screen as I pulled over to the side of the road:

- Location: City Centre
- Response: Code 3
- Type: Unconscious, cardiac arrest
- Call source: Person on scene
- Units: 90A1,25A2
- Remarks:
  - 14 day old found unresponsive, blue, not breathing, no pulse
  - Fire is responding

I said: "Hey Joe, it's a Code 3 call and I will be pushing it...do you want to come up front?"

Joe replied: "No, that's OK, I'll stay back here."

I said "OK, buckle up."

I quickly entered the address in the second GPS unit we had. Then, I flipped on the switches to activate the emergency lights and strobes, and looked out for traffic. It was morning, with people heading to work, so traffic was steady. I turned on the siren and began a U-turn, slowly waiting for traffic to stop. I spun around and gunned the engine; the engine roared as it picked up speed.

We were at least eight to ten minutes away from this call, and if it was real, this infant needed immediate resuscitation and a hospital. I drove faster than usual to this call, ensuring that I stopped at all red lights, as usual. We didn't need to get into a crash. I found that alternating the phasor with the hyper yelp siren seemed to get people's attention better at intersections.

I called our Dispatch on route: "25A2."

Dispatch: "25A2."

I said: "25A2, is ALS on scene yet?"

Dispatch: "25A2, affirmative. 90A1 is on scene."

Over the radio, I could hear Dispatch having a conversation: "90A1 do you require ITT from Children's?"

90A1: "Negative, but it's a viable arrest."

Hearing this confirmed that they needed our help. I pushed the gas pedal down. Now I was going faster than I would normally have on a Code 3 run. I could feel the adrenalin rush through my body. Although I was used to driving Code 3 from all these years, this was a serious call and seconds counted, so I pushed it a bit on this run.

As we approached the scene, I could see the advanced life support ambulance and the fire truck parked on the street with their emergency lights flashing. I pulled right up in front of the ALS car. As I exited, I could smell the brakes from all the hard stops en route to the scene. I headed toward the side door of the ALS car; it was open, and a firefighter was standing outside. There were a couple more firefighters nearby and one was entering the house. I entered the back of the ALS car and as soon as I was inside I could see a very small infant on the stretcher; a firefighter was doing compressions with his hands wrapped around the infant's back and with both thumbs on the chest. One of the ALS paramedics was at the back adjusting the cardiac monitor, and the second ALS was ventilating the infant with a BVM.

The ALS paramedic (Jim) said: "Hey Luch, can you come over and take over bagging?"

I replied: "Sure."

Jim said: "I need an airway; find the smallest one you can find." I looked in the cabinet, found a small black one, and looked at it; it was clearly too big. I rummaged around in the stack of airways all wrapped in plastic. Finally, I saw a pink one. It was tiny and looked like it would work, so I tore open the package and handed it to Jim to insert. He tried to insert it and, as if I read his mind, I began looking for a tongue depressor as he said: "I need a tongue depressor." Just then, I handed him one. He had a small grin on his face as he took it.

I looked up at the ALS paramedic at the monitor (Doug). He looked over and said: "Hi Luch. We are working this but we don't have a time down, and (the infant) was found pulseless and no respirations, blue." I looked down at the infant. It looked just like the infant resuci dolls we practice on — almost identical actually — same size, and lifeless.

Doug began to drill in the infant's left leg to insert an IO (intraosseous) IV site. He was having trouble gaining access.

Jim moved out of the way and said: "OK, move in, I'm going to try to intubate." I began to squeeze the small bag, looking for chest rise between the firefighter doing compressions. I looked at the firefighter who was tirelessly compressing the tiny chest.

I said: "Hi, are you OK? Do you need a break?"

He replied: "No, I'm good." Jim said: "Is the air getting into the chest?"

The firefighter said: "I can feel the chest rise as he vents" (meaning as I bagged the infant).

Jim moved in with a straight blade laryngoscope and a tiny ET tube. I hyperventilated the infant prior to his attempt. He moved in and could see he was having difficulty visualizing the chords as he struggled to insert the tube. It was a failed attempt and I moved back in to ventilate the infant. My partner (Joe) had his head poked in through the side door as did the Fire Captain who was standing beside him. Doug, who was still trying to get an IO access, said: "Jim looks like this one is not good. Going to try another site."

Jim made three attempts to intubate and on the third try was successful. I held the tube as it was taped in place. Jim said: "I know I don't have to remind you, but for god's sake do not let go of that tube." I nodded and said: "I got it". Doug, who had finally got the IO inserted and IV running, had already done the calculations for drug dosages for the cardiac arrest and had initiated the first course. There was some discussion with the Fire Captain about who was coming in the Amb with us to the hospital; it was decided that the infant's mother was going to be in the back with us as we transported to the hospital.

My partner initially was going to take over venting the infant as he was not VPOP so could not drive Code 3 to the hospital, but just before we were ready to leave our duty superintendent arrived and said she would drive us in. The same firefighter was continuing with compressions; I vented the infant every three to four compressions, and Doug managed the monitor and drugs.

We were ready to depart for the hospital, with the crying mother sitting in the back, the firefighter doing chest compressions, me bagging, and Doug watching the monitor. Jim, who was attending, was overseeing everything and said: "Can anyone think of anything else we have not done that we could be doing?" Nobody said anything. We felt the Ambulance move and the siren wail as we slowly and smoothly moved away from the curb. I looked down at the infant, who was still looking lifeless, but now with some colour due to the CPR in progress. We had to suction the ET tube en route as there was blood coming up during compressions. When we arrived at the trauma centre, I walked out as the stretcher was pulled out slowly, keeping my hand on the ET tube at all times and squeezing a small amount of air into the lungs as I went. In the trauma room there was staff everywhere, as well as a portable infant bed with a heat system to keep the infant warm. Jim began giving a verbal report to the staff after we entered. An ER physician came up to me and asked if the tube was in place; they wanted to auscultate the lungs to verify placement. Soon after, we excited the trauma room with the stretcher.

When we exited, the Superintendent who drove us in said: "CIS has been called. Do any of you need anything? A break, have a coffee?"

I looked at my partner who knew I wanted to have a coffee before this whole thing started. So, I said: "Sure, we will grab a coffee and then be good to go."

The Superintendent said: "I will put you out of service. Take the time you need." I replied: "OK sure, thanks."

We left in our Amb and headed to the Starbucks just a few blocks away. As we drank our coffee, the events of the call continued to process inside my head: the visuals, the sound, the voices of all the people involved in the call. It was a blur and my brain was processing it. I did not feel sad or upset, just a state of transition that often happens to me after intense high energy calls. My partner and I talked a bit about the call but did not discuss details as he was also processing the call. For some of our coffee break we sat in silence just processing and absorbing.

After we finished our coffee, we climbed back into the car, called Dispatch, and put us back in service. A moment later the CAD blipped: another Code 3 call.

Chest pain....or is it?

I was driving a shift, when we got a call for a forty-seven-year-old female who was apparently having chest pain. It was a layered call with FD and ALS. We were dispatched Code 3 and were first on the scene, but had some difficulty gaining access to the twelve-story apartment building. It was a very nice building — it was polished, and obviously an expensive building. We were finally able to gain access, and brought the stretcher, the O2, and our kit. When we rolled up to the apartment door, we knocked, and in a few moments a woman in her late forties opened the door; she was bent over and almost crawling on the floor. My partner glanced back at me, and I gave a raised eyebrow.

He said: "Hi, are we here for you?"

The woman replied, "Yes," then let out a groaning sound. She half crawled, half walked toward the living room area. Carrying the O2, I followed behind my partner, John, who was carrying the kit. As we followed her, John asked: "What seems to be the problem this evening?"

The woman replied: "Ohhhh, I can't breathe, ohhh....."

She made her way to the foam mattress in the living room. John interjected just as she made it there and said: "I will need you to sit down so I can access you. Sit on the couch over here." I noticed the TV was on and the news was broadcasting some violence over-seas.

The woman stopped and groaned as she walked hunched over to the couch, laid back, put her feet up on the arm rests, and crossed her feet.

After putting the O2 tank down, I asked: "Where would we find your care card and medications?" She replied: "Oh, I have my card over on the table, and the medications are there also."

I replied: "OK, I see them thanks." I grabbed my radio mike and called Dispatch: "23A, you can cancel Fire."

Dispatch replied: "10-4."

John said: "So you said you are feeling short of breath?"

The patient replied, "Yes," and touched her chest. I observed her breathing effort and it was normal: Her breaths per minute were approximately 18-20, she had good colour, and she was clearly not experiencing SOB that required any type of intervention. I had been looking over the meds and found Clonazepam, Lorazepam, and Cipralex. I handed them over to John as he continued with his questions.

John said: "Do you have any chest pain?"

The patient replied: "Yes a little bit."

John went through a series of questions to decide if he believed it was ischemic chest pain and if we still required ALS, which was en route, Code 3. John asked the patient: "Does it radiate? What is the severity from a scale of 0-10 if 0 is no pain and 10 is excruciating pain? Have you ever had this pain before? When did the pain start? Is the pain sharp or dull? Does the pain move or radiate anywhere? Does the pain get worse if you take a deep breath in? What were you doing when the pain started? Have you taken anything for the pain?"

The patient replied: "No, the pain does not radiate. It's about a 3 out of 10. Yes, I have when I was in my homeland in Israel. It started 2 days ago, when I started packing for my trip; I leave tomorrow morning. No, the pain does not move anyplace. I was just watching the news when the pain started. No, the pain does not get worse when I take in a deep breath. I took ASA when I called 911.; they told me to take 4."

John completed a set of vitals (BP, Pulse, O2 Sat, RR) and asculated her chest. He then turned to me and said: "You can cancel ALS." I grabbed my radio mike and called Dispatch: "23A, you can cancel ALS please."

Dispatch: "23A, 10-4. 88A1 did you copy the cancel?"

88A1responded: "10-4."

Just then, the fire department entered the residence. I turned to them and said: "Hey, sorry guys, we would have cancelled you but we didn't know you were on this one."

John continued with his questions: "So, it sounds like you are having an anxiety attack. Have you experienced them before?"

The patient replied: "Yes, I have had them before."

John said: "How are you feeling now?"

The woman replied: "Feeling much better, thank you."

John said: "Did you want to come to the hospital for a check-up this evening?"

The woman said: "Well, what do you think?"

John: "Well, I am not a doctor. My job is to take people to the hospital, so really it is up to you if you want to go."

The woman replied: "No, I think I am fine. Was just feeling stressed from the news."

I said: "Yes, keep the news off. It will just make you more anxious."

John said: "Is there anything else we can do for you this evening?"

The patient replied: "No, I will be fine."

John said: "OK, we are just going to get you to sign our form before we leave."

I already had the form filled out with the spot marked for her to sign and had it opened on the flip page. I handed it to John and he motioned for her to sign. The woman signed the form, we loaded everything onto our cot, and headed down the elevator.

John said: "I tell you, I normally would insist on taking her, but clearly she was having an anxiety attack." I replied: "Oh, yeah, I totally agree. I would have done the same thing."

We loaded the equipment back in the car and I pulled away from the door of the building. I said: "I'm going to grab a bite to eat from my lunch before we clear." John replied: "Sure sounds good." After a short fifteen-minute food break, I hit clear on the CAD and in a few moments it sounded: "Blip...blip...blip."

I said: "Good thing I ate...knew we would get tagged with another call."

Head—on Collision

We had literally just got back to our station in the metropolitan area of Vancouver when the phone rang. I picked it up and the voice on the other end said: "You have a pre-alert on your CAD"; it was our dispatcher.

I replied "OK," and hung up the phone.

For the benefit of my partner, Bill, who had just walked into the washroom, I said out loud: "Hey, we have a pre-alert. I'm going to acknowledge it. See you outside."

I heard his voice from the washroom: "OK."

I walked outside and climbed into the driver's seat as I was driving tonight. I spun the CAD toward me, activated the 'Screen On' button (that illuminates the CAD screen), and read the details:

- Location: Intersection of Station Rd. and Kingsgate Ave
- Response: Code 2
- Type: MVA – 2 Car head-on
- Call source: Person on scene
- Units: 23A
- Remarks: Unknown number of pts, unknown injuries, unknown number of vehicles involved.

Bill, jumped in the attendant seat beside me and said: "What have we got?"

I replied: "It's an MVA. Pretty close so we should be able to clear if no injuries and make it back to get off on time for a change."

Bill said: "Roger that."

I pulled away onto the busy Kingsgate Ave. All the morning rush hour traffic was heading to work. Normally that means a bunch of sleepy, rushed and impatient commuters, but on this day the traffic was flowing well. As we approached within a block of the accident location, I expected the traffic to slow, but it didn't.

I said: "This is odd. Normally there would be backed-up traffic at this point because it is in the middle of the intersection apparently."

Bill replied: "Yeah, no kidding. It is odd."

We pulled right up to the intersection and, to my disbelief, there was in fact a two-vehicle head-on collision in the middle of it. Three people were standing outside of their vehicles, there were no four-way flashers on, and traffic was driving around the accident scene as if it was not even there. I found this very profound.

I activated all my emergency lights, and hit the siren for a short yelp, waiting for traffic to stop. I moved into the intersection parallel to the two vehicles. I looked over to the people standing talking among the vehicles that had collided. There was nobody inside any of the vehicles. I picked up the radio mike and said: "23A."

Dispatch: "23A."

I said: "23A, cancel any other medical resources to this call."

Dispatch: "10-4."

My partner had already left the Amb and I could see him talking to the people near the collision. I carefully opened my door and, as I stepped out, vehicles were zooming past me very closely, driving around the Ambulance as they were going straight through the intersection. They seemed to be oblivious that both lanes were now blocked by us and the two vehicles in the accident. I carefully walked to the front of the Ambulance as vehicles wizzed by within only a few feet of the Ambulance. Just then, a FD pumper truck arrived and blocked the other side of the two vehicles in the collision. I grabbed my portable radio mike and said: "23A, we are going to require the Code 5s Code 3 for traffic control before there is another accident here."

Dispatch: "10-4. Will advise the Code 5." I noticed the FD had begun placing traffic cones along the roadway facing the front of the Ambulance to stop traffic from driving the other direction.

I moved back toward my door, cars still zooming past very fast and close. By now, I was getting pissed off! I didn't want to get hit! I grabbed the road flares – there were three in a plastic tube – and began lighting them and placing them on the road, adding to our emergency lights to ward off the flow of traffic driving around us.

It didn't work! Vehicles continued to drive past us, almost running over the flares! 'Geez' I thought, 'what is wrong with these people? Can't they just understand they have to divert around the block to avoid this intersection and carry on with their route?'

Bill came walking over and said: "I thought something was burning and noticed the flares."

I replied: "Well, wanted to do something before there is another accident. It's not working. I am going to move the car perpendicular to this accident scene to block traffic until the police get here."

I moved the Ambulance and adjusted the road flares, but vehicles were still moving around to the front of the Ambulance into oncoming traffic. 'This is nuts,' I thought. 'What the hell is wrong with these people?!'

I noticed a police car arrive. Two officers got out, put on their patrol jackets, with no safety vests. I walked over to the edge of the laneway, and shouted: "There are no injuries, we can clear. We just waited for you to arrive to take over traffic control. This intersection is crazy busy." The officer nodded and said: "Yes it's a busy intersection." He and his partner slowly walked over to talk to the drivers involved in the accident. I thought: 'What?? They are not going to take control of traffic?'

I looked over at Bill he shouted to me: "We are clear. Let's get out of here?" I noticed the FD were removing their traffic cones. I replied: "You got it! Let's get out of here."

I jumped in, turned on the siren, cleared the intersection, and headed back to the station, turning off my emergency equipment once we were in the regular traffic lanes.

As we drove back Bill said: "What a nightmare!!"

I replied: "You think? Geez and what was up with the cops? They certainly didn't take it seriously, and only one unit responded? I called for the 5s Code 3 for traffic and they send one unit?"

Bill replied: "You called? So did I from the cell phone, and they had the gall to ask me why we needed them Code 3."

I said: "You're kidding? OK, that is BS. When we are on scene if we need the police Code 3, they send them, period."

We drove the last few blocks back to the station in silence.

Wait for the police

My partner and I were at another station getting stock and doing some administration on the computers when the phone rang.

I answered: "23A."

The dispatcher on the phone said: "Hey, I have a pre-alert for you."

I replied, "OK, we are on it," hung up the phone, and headed downstairs where my partner was in the Unit Chief's office on the computer.

I said: "We have a pre-alert. I'll go out and acknowledge the call while you finish up."

My partner (Doug) replied: "OK, be right out."

I hopped in the attendant side of the cab, spun the CAD, and looked at the call. It was routine for an eighty-seven-year-old male with new onset of immobility. Basically he previously could move around but now could not, so called 911. Could be anything. I acknowledged the call and a few moments later the CAD sounded: "Blip...blip...blip."

I looked at the CAD, but the previous call was cancelled and a new call was now displayed on the CAD. This one read:

Code 3 for a possible overdose of cough syrup

32 yo female, history of mental health issues

I thought about this for a moment: 'Yup, seems to fit,' I thought.

I tapped the siren for a moment to get Doug out, now that it was a Code 3 call. I noticed Doug walking out as the CAD again sounded: "Blip...blip...blip." Another call came across the screen:

- Time: 2212
- Location: 522 Anyplace Street Vancouver
- Response: Code 3
- Type: Diabetic – Hypoglycemia (known history)
- Call source: Person on scene
- Units: 23A
- Remarks:
  - **Wait for police**
  - Aggressive Pt has a history of being aggressive when glucose levels are low

Doug climbed into the driver's seat and I said: "Well there have been three calls since the original. Looks like we are going to a diabetic call, Code 3." Doug spun the CAD around and read the call: "Aggressive... wait for the police..."

I said: "I know...I was thinking the same thing: this guy is aggressive due to low sugar, not because he is aggressive in general. What are the police going to do, wait until he is restrained? He needs his sugar brought up asap."

Doug replied: "Yup, I say we just go in if the police are not on scene." He pulled out and activated the emergency lights and siren.

I replied: "I agree. We just go in, assess the situation, and if there is something we can't handle we can back out. Fire will probably be on scene anyway."

Doug replied: "Agreed. This is stupid that they want us to wait for a hypoglycemic patient. Bunch of untrained call takers have no idea."

We continued on to the call. Traffic was fairly light as it was late evening. When we pulled up to the call there was a smaller (four-door crew-cab pickup) fire rescue truck on scene.

As we both got out of the Amb, I yelled to the firefighter standing outside of his truck and said: "We're going in; this is a diabetic patient. Follow us in if you want." The firefighter just looked a me, a bit stunned by my announcement.

As I proceeded around to the side of the Amb, a police car pulled up. I grabbed our kit and as the two officers got out of the car, I said: "We are not waiting, we are going in. This is a diabetic patient. He needs treatment. If you can follow us in that would be great." One of the officers, a male, replied: "Ah...sure."

We approached a home with a very manicured green area and proceeded around to the side of the house as we were told it was a rental residence we were responding to. As we approached the side door an East Indian man in his late 50s was standing there holding a glass filled with what looked like orange juice. The man said: "He is inside." I replied: "OK, thanks."

We entered the room and noticed a man lying on a bed in the living room area. He was on his back and was moving about and making some incomprehensible noises. From time to time, he would suddenly shake and thrash around. The two police officers and three firefighters were also in the room just behind us. My partner approached the patient.

I turned to the man who let is in and said: "How do you know this man?"

The man replied: "He is my tenant."

I said: "Is this how he acts when his sugar gets low?"

The man replied: "Yes, I have seen it a few times. I tried to give him some juice, but he would not drink it. We also made him a sandwich." He motioned to a sandwich on a plate. I began to open our kit and begin assembling the glucometer to test his blood sugar.

I said: "OK, thanks. Did you call 911?"

The man replied: "Yes, we could hear him screaming out."

We began talking to the patient and obtained a blood glucose reading of 1.7 mmol. It was very low, as we normally treat patients with any sugar reading less than 4.0mmol.

I said to Doug: "Do you see any veins where we can get a line?"

Doug replied: "I think I see some here. Need a tourniquet."

I handed Doug a rubber band tourniquet as I assembled the D10W (Dextrose 10% in water). He managed to get a 20G IV in the man's arm and we began administering the D10W, squeezing the bag to get the flow going faster. We had to control his arm, so he would not pull out his IV. There was a firefighter and my partner controlling his arm. The police looked on with concern but did not intervene as we had asked them to stand back unless needed.

After about 100ml of the D10W ran through, the patient began to calm down and was making eye contact, but was not yet responding to my partner's questions. After another few minutes and 50ml of IV the patient began responding to questions, slowly at first. You could tell he was dazed and confused. The low blood sugar affects the brain's ability to function and a person's cognitive functions are decreased.

I did another check of his glucometer reading and it was now 10.1mmol. I stopped the IV flow as we did not want his blood sugar to spike.

I said: "So John (patient) do you remember what happened?"

John replied: "Well, um, I remember having something to eat at some point, but I gave myself more insulin than normal."

I said: "Oh, why would you just give yourself more than directed by your doctor?"

John replied: "Well, it's just I was feeling a bit off so decided to make adjustments on my own."

I said: "Well, you know you should not make any adjustments to your insulin without your doctor directly advising you. Your sugar was very low — 1.7 — and you were combative. If we did not arrive when we did you could have dropped into a coma."

John replied: "Yeah, I know."

One of the police officers said to John: "This is like Jekyll and Hyde...I have never seen this before. One minute you were not responding and aggressive, and after some of that IV you are a pleasant calm man." As he said this, the officer shook his head side to side.

After this, I explained to the patient that we wanted to take him to the hospital, but over a thirty-minute discussion he continually refused. John said he would eat something and follow-up with his doctor and would stop self-administering extra insulin on his own without his doctor advising him so.

We packed up our equipment and left the residence. It was not surprising that the patient did not want to come to the hospital; most diabetics refuse further treatment once we give them sugar and wake up. There is nothing we can do about that. Also, I don't blame them — the hospital will just do some tests and release them in a few hours and tell them to follow-up with their family doctor.

We departed the scene, and as soon as Doug hit the 'Clear' button on our CAD, another call popped up...just another normal non-stop night in the city.

Sometimes it's better not to drink...other times it is

It was early evening and I was attending, as I had a paramedic student with me. My regular partner was off for the block, so I had a different partner every day this block. At times this was challenging, as when you work with someone on a regular basis you get into a routine, know what to expect from your partner, and calls go very seamlessly when it comes to each other's roles. Adding a paramedic student to the mix places a higher load onto the preceptor. Fortunately, my call-in partner was very experienced, and we worked well together.

My student was a bit weak on his confidence but was very keen and motivated. He still needed one competency – a spinal immobilization. Without completing all the required competencies, students cannot write their licensing exam; passing would grant them a Paramedic license and allow them to work. However, I do not focus my precepting on their competencies, and prefer that they are capable of performing the job at a basic level within their skill set independently. It is most important that they are able to conduct a thorough assessment, know how to make critical decisions, and above all else don't do any harm to their patients. It takes at least two years of high-volume calls to really get the experience necessary to walk into virtually any call and feel comfortable managing it. Every call is different, so being able to adapt to the constantly changing environments is essential. Experience takes time — there is no short-cut.

We were driving in our response area after having cleared a call recently when the CAD sounded: "Blip...blip...blip."

I spun the CAD around and looked at the call:

- Response: Code 3
- Call Source: Person at scene
- Type: Long Fall > 15ft
- Units: 23A, 37A1
- Remarks:
  - Security witness man fall 20-30ft after climbing over a fence.
  - Possible intoxication
  - Police at scene
  - FD responding

I spun the CAD toward my partner and said: "It's a long fall in Anytown. Just head toward the Cross Gate Mall off of Parallel Road. I will put it in the GPS for you."

My partner looked at the call briefly and said: "OK, that would be great. I will head in that direction."

I entered the information into the GPS. It was early morning (around 2:00am), raining, and the traffic was very light. My partner entered the freeway and the posted speed limit was 100kmph on the highway, but she was driving slower than the posted speed limit. I looked over at a tow truck passing us in the HOV lane as we sped toward the call, Code 3. I was almost going to suggest to my partner that if we are going below the posted speed limit that we shut it down; there was no reason to have our lights and siren wailing if vehicles were passing us. Just then, she flipped off all the emergency lights and turned the siren off. I said: "I was just going to suggest that." She replied: "Well, I am not going to get us killed driving fast in this rain to get to this call." I didn't reply, but thoughts drifted in my mind that if she was not capable of driving an emergency vehicle in a bit of rain with confidence then perhaps she should not be a Paramedic. It was a bid of a run and we arrived to find the FD and ALS unit, as well as the PD on scene.

We got out and headed over with our jump bag and stretcher. There was a gathering of emergency personnel below a high concrete wall that ended at the top of an upper parking lot adjacent to an apartment building. The rain had lessened now. As we approached I noticed about three firefighters lingering about fifteen feet from the patient. There was a female ALS paramedic speaking to them, or, rather, shouting very erratically something about not spinaling the patient. I instructed my student to get over to the patient to assist as required. The second ALS paramedic was with the patient and a firefighter was attempting to hold C-spine. The patient was moving about and resisting the C-spine control.

The male ALS paramedic (Doug) was getting frustrated. We began sliding the clam shell (ROS) underneath the man. I found out that he had jumped from the top of the upper parking lot (twenty-five to thirty feet in height) and landed in the plants and firm soil. He did not lose consciousness as far as we knew. There were no obvious injuries to the man, but he was intoxicated with alcohol. There were only four of us working to secure the clam shell, although any more hands would have probably gotten in the way. At one point the man's legs came up and almost kicked me in the head as I attempted to secure his torso and legs to the clam. I yelled out, "Someone grab his legs now!! He just about kicked me in the head," a bit pissed off actually that the three cops and four other firefighters were not helping restrain the man as we struggled to secure him. Two cops jumped in finally to hold his legs down. The other female paramedic (Jill) was yelling from fifteen feet away that we should sedate the man or not C-spine him as he was being combative.

Her partner (Doug) said: "We have to C-spine him we have no choice. He has had a long fall and we can't sedate him due to possible head injury." He was very frustrated with all of this. I could not believe Jill was interacting with her partner this way and second-guessing him during his treatment. I knew Doug and he was a very experienced ALS Paramedic.

We finally strapped the man onto the clam shell and secured his head and hands. He calmed down a bit and was not struggling as much. After arriving at the Emergency Room, the ER Physician ordered a CT scan to rule out intracranial hemorrhage. I stopped by the trauma bay approximately fifteen minutes after finishing my paperwork. The man was sitting up and had not had the CT yet. I walked over to him as I was leaving my paperwork for he ER nurse's chart.

I said to the patient: "Do you realize how lucky you are?"

The patient replied: "Yeah...I guess."

I said: "You jumped over twenty-five feet. You could have been seriously injured or killed, the only thing that saved you is that you are so intoxicated."

The patient replied: "Yeah, well good thing then." I shook my head and left the trauma room. Amazes me that people are so lucky and can barely perceive it.

Runny nose

We responded routine to a thirty-four-year-old Asian male who had a runny nose who was living in a basement suite. The student and my partner had taken the lead. We entered a typical illegal basement suite in the city; the ceilings were lower than normal and slanted on one end. Appliances were placed haphazardly in a mock kitchen.

I followed my partner with his student and they began to question the patient. The student said: "What seems to be the problem today sir?"

The patient said: "I have a runny nose, and it won't stop running."

The student, with a very concerned look on his face, said: "OK sir, how long has this been going on?"

The patient replied: "Oh maybe an hour or so, then I called. I don't know what to do."

My thoughts drifted to handing the patient a tissue and telling him 'we have real calls to do and suck it up or take some over-the-counter cold medication.' But we cannot say that and must transport anyone who calls us to the hospital, no matter how ridiculous it is.

My partner now intervened to get this call rolling: "OK, sir. We are going to take you up to the hospital to have the doctor check you out." My partner had the legal obligatory statement down pat from years of doing calls like this.

The patient said: "OK."

We walked the patient to the car that I had parked in the alley behind the house. It was a short, fourteen-minute drive to the hospital. The patient emerged from the back of the Ambulance with a tissue in his hand.

I thought 'My partner fixed the problem...gave him a tissue...lol.'

The patient was walked to the paramedic staging area inside the hospital. I was fortunate to not have to be the one to give the report to the triage nurse. Sometimes it's nice having drive day.

Mascara

We responded routine to a residence that was five minutes from the hospital. An Asian woman met us at the door and was complaining of being unable to open her eyes fully. She had gotten eyeliner tattoo earlier that day. She was able to walk to the Ambulance and to the triage area. My partner and his student put an ice pack on her eyes and she said: "Oh that feels better." Apparently, the tattoo artist did not explain fully that there would be swelling, and subsequent healing after the tattoo. After we got back into the Amb, I turned to my partner and said: "We can't make this stuff up...people just would not believe we get these types of calls." My partner, smiling now, replied, "Nope...we certainly can't," and laughed.

The Overdose

I worked my last night shift of my block. My regular partner had booked off and I knew he was going to be gone, but I still had my student who I was precepting. My partner for this shift was someone I had worked with before, but not often. We had a rather boring evening dealing with somewhat stupid Amb calls...until the early morning.

We attended a fifty-year-old female called in by her daughter who found her unconscious, unresponsive and barely breathing. We arrived in less than three minutes as we were very close to the call. On arrival, we found a female on the floor, unresponsive, and GCS 3. My student had a tough time inserting an OPA, so my partner forced it in. The patient's SPO2 was 66% and she was breathing at a rate of four breaths per minute. After moving furniture in the dimly light room to gain access, we began resuscitation. As my student used the BVM and bagged the patient, my partner took a blood sugar. Meanwhile, the daughter told us that her mother had used cocaine and was a regular user. The woman had pinpoint pupils, decreased GCS and her respiration rate indicated an opiate OD.

I drew up 0.8 Narcan to administer IM. Due to the low light in the room, I had to use my flashlight to confirm the medication and dose. My partner confirmed a glucose of 16.7mmol so we ruled out a diabetic concern. Luckily, my student was able to vent the patient and increase her SPo2 to 98% on 100% via BVM. I handed my partner the Narcan syringe and she administered it into the patient's right arm IM. ALS (Advanced life support) arrived, we continued treatment, and the patient was transported to Burnaby hospital.

Upon coming to, the patient was confused, combative, and aggressive; she thought we were the police arresting her for something she did not do. The patient was admitted to the ER for further assessment and tests. Just another day on the job.

COPD

The last call of the night was of a COPD patient, fifty years of age. On arrival, the patient was sitting on the back of a Fire Department truck bumper with O2 at 10LPM via face mask. The patient was conscious and was breathing at a rate of 45+, but was unable to speak in full sentences and was constantly stating "I cannot breathe." I osculated with my scope and breath sounds were virtually absent, even though the patient was making extreme effort to breathe.

As we loaded the patient into our Ambulance, ALS arrived; I did not even know they had been dispatched (it's common that we are not informed). They began assessment and after the ALS Paramedic called a doctor for orders they began to vent the patient with a BVM and PEEP valve. I drove the ALS Amb and followed my partner Code 3 to RCH hospital.

When we arrived I opened the back doors. The ALS attendant was in the process of incubating the patient after giving Versed. There was blood coming from the ET tube and (luckily) after asking my student for safety glasses, there was spray from the ET tube that splattered my right arm. I told them not to worry, as I did not have any broken skin. We offloaded to the ER trauma bay, bagging the intubated patient on the way. After the call, we were out of service for cleaning, so we went to a nearby station for stocking and cleaning. My partner was concerned that we were going to get another call. I told her I was going to call Dispatch and put the Amb out so service, as I had been sprayed with blood and needed a uniform change.

Even though the blood did not actually touch my shirt to my knowledge, I was emotionally done. I was not capable of doing another call. We returned to the station and were off on time.

4x4 accident

I was working in a semi-rural area when the pagers sounded: "Beep beep beep....shhhhhhhhhhh...34 Kilo Code 3 call...34 Kilo Code 3... shhhhhhhhhhh."

I always jumped when the pagers sounded as they were so loud, annoying and contained static after the call. My partner (Tom) made the call to Dispatch to get the call info. Once he got off the phone he said: "We have a rollover down an embankment on Forest B Road, up in the area that everyone 4x4 and parties a lot." I replied: "How far up the road is it? That road is pretty rough and doing a spinal down that will suck." Tom replied: "Yeah, no kidding." We headed out to the car.

Once clear of the bay, Tom, who was driving, activated all the emergency equipment (emergency lights and siren), and I donned my ears (hearing protection), as the way they placed the sirens in these old Fords were brutally loud in the cab. My partner knew the way to the forest service road. It was raining steadily as we screamed to the call. It was later in the evening and getting dark; this was going to add to the challenges of the call. The RCMP were on the way, as were the Fire Department. We were over half an hour from this call, which was a long response if someone was seriously hurt, as takes time to extricate, package, assess and transport a patient to hospital.

Tom turned onto the Forest B Road, and had to slow down due to the potholes and ribbed areas of the road that made the entire vehicle shake and rattle. These ambulances were already rough enough on paved roads — let alone on back roads — due to their suspension. The road was muddy, wet, and slippery, but compact and firm, so there was no obvious chance of getting stuck. We continued up the road, our red and white lights and strobe lights flickering into the darkness as we went. We finally rounded a bend in the roadway and came upon two RCMP cruisers with their red and blue lights flashing. As we got out, donning our lime green issued rain parkas, one of the constables approached us to give us a report.

RCMP Officer 1: "Hi guys. Looks like the driver is pretty banged up. He is bleeding and walked up the bank by himself. His truck is about twenty feet down the embankment."

I replied: "Do you suspect he has been drinking?"

RCMP Officer 1: "Yes he definitely has, but he is still able to walk. He is leaning against the cruiser — refused to sit inside out of the rain." Tom and I walked over to the man without our equipment as he was only a short distance from the Amb. As I approached, I noticed he was holding a large dressing to the left side of his face; there was blood covered all over his face, and he had an obvious laceration to his head.

I said to him: "Hi my name is Luke. (I often use my son's name as my full name is too difficult for people to understand especially when they are hurt and disorientated) I'm a Paramedic (I always identify myself even though I'm in uniform, as when people are injured they often just see uniforms and what is obvious to us is not obvious to them). "I just want to check you out. What is your name?"

The man replied: "Wayne."

I replied; "OK, Wayne, looks like you have hit your head and have cut yourself up. Do you remember all the events leading up to the crash? Did you lose conscious at all?"

Wayne said: "No, not that I recall. Think I smashed my head on the door when it went over."

I said: "Were you wearing your seat belt? And do you have any neck pain?"

Wayne said: "Yeah, I was wearing my seat belt. I don't have any neck pain — just my head hurts bad, and I have this cut on my mouth."

I said: "I am just going to take a look at the wound to your face, so I need to move this bandage." I removed the partially blood-soaked bandage and when I did, I saw a hole in his left cheek the size of a loonie;

there was blood oozing out, and when I looked inside his mouth I could see the blood pooling in his mouth. Something told me he was not wearing his seat belt as he said. People often say they wore one, so the police do not ticket them, even though my only reason to find out is to help determine the possibility of potential injuries. I gave the patient the dressing to apply pressure again until I could place a new one over it.

Just then my partner arrived with a hard collar; I didn't have to ask Tom to get it as he knew from the mechanism of the accident that we had to spinal this man even though he walked up the bank. I wanted to get him inside the warm Ambulance as well. The rain had stopped now but the air was damp and cool.

I said: "Wayne we are just going to put his hard collar on your neck as a precautionary measure."

Wayne said: "Yeah OK, my mouth is really bleeding here man."

I replied: "Yes, I know, and I'm not sure if we will be able to stop it completely until you get to the hospital. We need to make sure we protect your neck. Sometimes you can have an injury that is not obvious."

We applied the hard collar, walked him the few feet back to the Amb, and placed him on the cot with the clam down. When we laid him on his back he began to complain about blood running down his throat and started coughing, as it was interfering with his airway. I tried to suction his airway but could not keep up, so I rolled him on his left side, wound down, to allow it to drain. I ended up using blankets and securing him on his left side down (lateral spinal) so he would not aspirate. Even on his left side the blood was still draining down his throat, causing some airway issues. I removed the dressing and let him cover the wound loosely with a larger abdominal pad on the spine board to catch the blood oozing out. There was no way to apply enough direct pressure to stop the bleeding. After we had secured him to the board, we were ready to go. I completed a set of vitals and removed the patient's wet clothing. I began setting up an IV.

Tom said: "Hey, I am going to get the cops to help me turn around. Let me know if you need me back here; I will try to give you the smoothest ride I can."

I replied: "Thanks Tom. It will be rough back here, but we have to get him to the hospital so just do your best…appreciate it."

As Tom turned the Ambulance around, it rocked side to side. I had to suction Wayne's mouth out every few minutes to keep the blood from running down his throat. Tom began our forty-minute trip down the road, although it had taken us twenty-two minutes to get to the scene in the first place. Taking his time, Tom was going as slow as he could to avoid jarring us in the back even though it was impossible to give us a smooth ride. Wayne's vitals were stable, but I still had Tom stop after ten minutes so I could insert a 18G IV catheter into Wayne's right arm vein.

Wayne was losing blood, and it was also possible that he had sustained internal injuries that his body was compensating for. Furthermore, there was also a possibility of a sudden change in BP; starting an IV on him was standard precaution for trauma patients to allow for IV access by the hospital and giving fluids if his vital signs changed en route to the hospital. I had packed gauze on the outside of his cheek, which blocked the hole in his cheek, but then the blood then pooled inside his cheek, causing it to run down his throat. I decided to remove the gauze and allow the blood to drain out the hole in his cheek onto a large abdominal dressing. By doing this, the blood was diverted from going down his throat. We continued to the hospital and on arrival we were quickly directed into one of the trauma rooms with staff awaiting our arrival.

Revenge

My partner Tim and I were in quarters when the hotline rang. Tim answered and after hanging up said: "We have a stabbing."

I replied: "A stabbing…oh." My mind processed this statement. This could be a simple, little wound or something serious. The area we covered ranged from common to serious stabbings and GSW (gunshot wounds). It was my partner's drive day, so I was attending — my turn to be on and make the critical treatment and transport decisions.

When we got into the car and looked at the CAD it showed a location only a few miles from us. We were close. It was also in an area that was known for a high population of homeless people and street drug users. Tim activated the lights and siren and aggressively drove toward the call. There was moderate traffic and it was mid-day. On the way to the call, the dispatcher told us of a MVA on the bridge we would be taking to the nearest trauma center.

My partner grabbed the mic and said: "Will we have access to get past the accident?"

The dispatcher replied: "We are not sure at this time. We don't have that information."

Tim hung up the mic and said: "That's great. Now we have no access and might have to go around to the other bridge." We arrived in a few minutes and noticed yellow police tape surrounding the scene. As we pulled up, we saw two firefighters beside a man on the roadway.

Tim said: "I'm just going to pull out and back in for access." My partner backed the Ambulance toward the firefighters, so we could have easier access to the patient with our cot and would be quicker to leave the scene. I looked over and noticed one firefighter (Firefighter 1) was applying pressure to the man's shoulder, while another (Firefighter 2) was using a BVM to ventilate the patient.

We were parked only thirty feet from the patient and after exiting the car I proceeded directly over to the patient to quickly assess what we needed to do. I opened the back doors of the car and removed the stretcher; I knew we would need to load him onto it quickly if it was serious. I did not bring my jump kit as the firefighters already had their kits on scene with O2, and anything I would be needing for treatments would be in the back of the car.

On approach, I noticed the man was stripped of clothing from the waist up. One firefighter was applying pressure to his right shoulder with a very large pile of dressings. Blood was still running down onto the roadway, creating a pool of blood the size of a large dinner plate.

The other firefighter was using a BVM. The firefighter at the BVM said: "The guy is breathing. We are just assisting his breaths."

I looked at the firefighter holding the dressings and said: "Have you seen the wound?"

The firefighter replied: "No, we didn't want to disturb the dressing in place."

I replied: "OK, keep holding pressure for now. Did you notice any other wounds?"

The firefighter at the BVM said: "No."

I scanned the body and moved down the man's legs one at a time, quickly looking for any other blood loss or instability. I reached for his radial pulse and found one, but it was very weak and rapid.

Just then, another firefighter brought more dressings over to the firefighter holding pressure on the wound. He applied more dressings on top and now there was a stack of dressings over three inches thick over the wound. My thoughts raced; I worried that there might be too many dressings and that the firefighter was able to apply enough pressure to stop the bleeding. We didn't have time for that now — this man was in critical condition and needed a trauma centre. We had to get him on the cot and in the back of our Amb immediately and begin heading to the trauma centre.

Tim arrived, and I said: "OK we need to fore and aft him onto the cot." To the firefighters I said: "OK, you guys keep bagging him and holding pressure. You" – I pointed to the firefighter holding pressure – "will continue doing that to the hospital."

Tim said, "I am going to set up an IV for you in the back of the car," and departed. Another firefighter and I lifted the patient 'fore and aft' onto the cot, while the other firefighter continued to hold pressure on the wound as we wheeled the patient toward and into the back of the car.

After loading the patient into the back of the Ambulance, I said to Tim: "Can you grab me two ABD dressings...you have clean gloves." We don't want to cross contaminate other equipment when we have possible blood or body fluids on our hands. Tim reached up, grabbed a couple of dressings, and handed them to me.

I said to the firefighter holding the dressing in place: "I am going to get you to remove all those dressings, so we can take a look at the wound and then reapply direct pressure with these dressings." The firefighter said: "OK, no problem" He removed the thick stack of dressings from the would that was still allowing blood to seep past, down his shoulder and onto the floor of the Ambulance. When the dressings were removed, I noticed two 4cm clean incisions: one was just above his clavicle and was not bleeding, and the second was below and more toward the man's neck and was bleeding profusely. I placed the two abdominal dressings in place and simultaneously the firefighter reapplied firm pressure on the shoulder. I looked back and noticed Tim had placed a tourniquet on the man's left arm and was looking for a vein to start an IV. He clearly needed an IV; but he needed a trauma room more.

I said: "Tim, don't worry about the IV. I will get in en route. He needs a trauma room...we need to get going now."

Tim said, "OK, let me know when you are ready to go," and left the back of the Ambulance, leaving the two firefighters with me. Firefighter 1 was holding pressure on the wound, and Firefighter 2 assisted in venting the patient.

I still had not obtained a BP from the patient and my BP cuff was in my kit which was not accessible, as Firefighter 2 was positioned over the cabinet. I decided not to use the cuff, as I did not want him to stop venting the patient and knew that the BP was not going to change the treatment of the patient or our destination; this patient was in critical condition. I could see the chest rise and the efforts of the patient to breathe. I checked the radial pulse and it was absent. I checked the carotid pulse and it was present and rapid (estimated at over 120 bpm).

Tim yelled out from the front of the cab: "Are you ready to go?"

I replied: "Yes, let's get going, thanks."

Tim began moving the Ambulance. As he did I started looking for IV access in the patient's left arm. Specifically, I was looking for one at his AC (antecubital), a typically large bifurcation of veins from the brachial that often is easy to access at the inner side of the elbow at the bend. This is known as a trauma access site. Normally we will look for

IV access at the hands and move toward the upper arm. The rationale is that if we miss getting a start we have to move up to a farther vein site. If we blow the AC then there is not much farther we can go, so getting it right the first time is very important, and since when we start IVs on patients at this location that are often in very poor condition, blowing an IV is not an option. The pressure on the person starting the IV is even higher. I heard a second siren behind us and looked through the back window; it was an RCMP cruiser. Since this was a stabbing and a possible crime, the police had to either accompany us in the back with the patient or follow us to the hospital and stay with the patient at all times as part of their investigation.

I went back to my task of looking for IV access. I re-tightened the tourniquet and the patient's vein popped out at the AC site, but not as pronounced as I would have liked, since I was planning on inserting a 16g IV catheter. (16g is a larger size that will allow higher volumes of fluid as the needle is larger; the smaller the number, the larger the bore of IV. I would have considered a 14g but did not want to take the chance of blowing the vein, as his BP was low. Also, a 16g will deliver a large volume of fluids very quickly and even faster if we attached a pressure infuser). I organized all my supplies and equipment: tegaderm (thin plastic clear film placed over the IV after insertion), medical tape, gauze, interlock device, primed IV tubing (already done for me by Tim), alcohol wipes, and a 16g catheter.

As Tim drove, there were bumps in the road. He was doing his best, but the back was still swaying from side to side. I did not want to have him stop to insert the IV but there is a risk that the minute you begin inserting the IV the Ambulance hits a bump and the IV is missed — not a good scenario. The pressure on me to get this right just increased. Also, as per our treatment guidelines, we are supposed to stop the Ambulance when inserting IVs for safety and proficiency. In this case, seconds counted, and I had to use my judgement to make the best choice under the circumstances. I opened the 16g IV catheter, spun the plastic catheter (they tend to stick and not advance properly if we don't). I had already swabbed the area, so I looked out the front window to see the traffic pattern and plan when there was smooth road. Sometimes we will call out to our partner who is driving and say: "I'm doing a start make it as smooth as you can" or "Let me know when you are at a light, I want to do a start."

Today I was just going to go for it. Tim was busy concentrating on driving and I did not want to distract him anymore. I picked my time, stabilizing my right hand on the patient's arm, as I held his arm straight with my left. I inserted the needle, advanced it slowly another 4mm, and I saw a flash (blood will fill a small chamber in the IV catheter confirming entry into a vein). I flattened the IV slightly and, using my index finger, began advancing the plastic catheter smoothly. Just then, we hit a small bump...but my hand was stable on the patient's arm and everything just moved together and my needle placement did not move...fortunately. I completed the insertion and retracted the needle back into the IV catheter safety chamber until it locked. I pressed down on the back plastic portion with my right thumb as I released the tourniquet. I held it tight on his skin as we had hit another bump and I did not want to lose it. I applied pressure 1-2cm above the insertion site with my middle and ring fingers of my right hand (it is like a little dance with your fingers, holding pressure simultaneously). I grabbed the IV tubing and twisted the end off the line with the index fingers and thumb of my right hand as I held pressure on the skin above the IV site. I held the IV tubing between my fingers in my left hand as I used my thumb and index finger of my right hand to twist off the IV plastic end. I knew there would be some blood seepage, using a 16g IV and at the AC site the blood wants to squirt out immediately. I continued to push firmly down above the insertion site with my right hand and, as soon as the plastic portion was removed, I dropped it on the floor. Blood began to seep out of the catheter hub, but very little as I had firm pressure above on the vein, stopping most of it. I inserted the IV line, turned it and locked it in place. I released the pressure above the insertion site and held the IV tubing with my right thumb and index finger as I reached over and opened the flow adjuster on the line to see if the line was patent. (If the IV had gone interstitial, the skin around the IV site would begin to fill with IV solution rather than going into the vein as intended and I would have to discontinue and find another site). The IV was good; there was a stream of flow in the drip chamber below the IV bag. I placed the tegaderm over the IV and placed several large pieces of tape to secure the IV in place.

I looked up at the patient and two firefighters and said: "I don't even know your guys' names; my name is Luciano."

Firefighter 1 smiled and said: "My name is Scott."

A moment later Firefighter 2 said: "My name is Alex."

I said: "Great, well how is the bagging going?"

Alex replied: "It's going well, no resistance."

I said: "OK, let me know if it changes." I looked at Scott: "How is the bleed?"

Scott replied: "It has stopped now that we took off that stack of dressings."

I said: "Good to hear."

My mind began processing what to do next. We were going to meet up with ALS (Advanced Life Support) very soon on the way to the trauma centre. I stood up and began looking in the medication section of the Ambulance, looking for TXA (trans eschimic acid). This was large vial of 10cc (1000mg) of a drug that is used to help support blood clotting with trauma patients with blood loss. I rummaged around and could not find it.

I yelled up toward Tim: "Hey Tim...where do you keep the TXA?"

Tim replied: "It's in the medication area on the shelf."

I said: "I can't find it. Are you sure it's kept there?"

Tim yelled back: "Yes, it should be there in the back."

I looked again, getting a bit frustrated as I could not find it. I could not locate it and thought that the ALS car would have some in their kits, so I could always use theirs. I took a look over at the patient: IV running, pressure on wound, assisted vents. Not much more I could do except do vitals and my BP cuff was in my kit. (I had asked my U/C to get us a second one to use in the back of the car during calls, but one had to be ordered and had not come in yet.)

Tim yelled out: "We are just pulling up with ALS."

He stopped, the side and back doors opened, and two familiar faces entered the back of the Ambulance. There were now three paramedics and two firefighters in the back; things were getting cramped very quickly. The ALS crew was working de-paired, meaning that the second paramedic and driver was a PCP not ALS, and typically assisted the ALS paramedic with tasks such as connecting the monitor, drawing up IV drugs, and preparing equipment. The second paramedic (Newman) began organizing the cardiac leads as the ALS (Paul) came beside me.

I said: "We have to get going guys; this guy is in rough shape."

Newman replied: "Someone has to get out and drive our car."

I said: "I'm not going anywhere."

Paul replied: "Guess you are going to have to drive our car in Newman." Newman looked up and paused a moment. I could tell he was not happy to have to leave the patient.

Newman said "OK," and exited the Ambulance. Shortly after he exited and closed the door, Tim began driving again. Paul looked over at me and asked: "What do we have?"

I replied: "We have a man with two stab wounds to his upper shoulder area. One is not bleeding. The one below the clavicle was bleeding profusely at first and I'm thinking is his subclavian artery. After we removed the stack of bulk dressings and replaced them with two, the bleed is under control. He was breathing on his own on arrival of the Fire Department and they were assisting when we arrived. He was found down unresponsive GCS of three. I have a 16G IV and have 400 cc infused. I have not been able to get a pressure yet. He has no radial pulses, but his carotid is present. There are no other stab wounds that we could find. I wanted to start TXA, but I can't find ours."

Paul took a moment, then said: "OK, good. Let's connect the monitor, get a pressure, and see what is happening. I called the trauma centre and told them to be ready; I knew you would be dealing with a shit show."

I replied: "Thanks. I did not have time to call. Tim called via Dispatch, I think, also." We both began connecting the basic five leads to get a rhythm and pulse rate. I placed the red and white foot leads as Paul placed the chest and arm leads. I looked at the monitor and the rhythm showed tachycardia rate, but good rhythm. The rate was 138 bpm, and Spo2 was 96%. I reached to check the man's femoral artery. I palpated and could not detect it.

I said: "I can't find his femoral." Paul reached over and felt for the patient's carotid and said: "I have his carotid. It's weak but present."

We continued to the trauma centre. When we arrived, we had to unload the patient with Scott holding pressure and Alex continuing to assist in ventilations as we moved as a unit through the doors. Paul had told me he had called and let the trauma room know we would be bringing in a guy in bad shape and to have a team ready for us. The PCC (Patient Care Co-ordinator) called out to us as she saw us enter and shouted out: "Trauma 2". I replied: "OK, thanks."

We entered, passed through the automatic trauma room doors, and entered the newly renovated and very brightly lit room. There was a team of staff wearing yellow protective gowns, gloves and face plastic face shields. I recognized one of the ER doctors and, as we approached the trauma table, I began talking.

I said: "We have a forty-six-year-old man who has sustained two stab wounds to the upper chest and shoulder area. One stab wound is not bleeding; the second was bleeding profusely and is now controlled with direct pressure. He was unconscious on arrival, has a carotid pulse, but we were not able to obtain his femoral. We checked his back and limbs and he does not have any other wounds. His vital signs are: Sats were 98% on 15 lpm; his pulse is 132, very weak at the carotid; and we were unable to get an accurate BP. We have been assisting his ventilations en route, have a 16G IV at the AC, and have infused a total of 800cc. We administered 8cc of TXA 1 cc every minute during transport."

When I finished, the ER doctor said: "Thanks." He began instructing staff on things he wanted done, even though everyone was already doing various things automatically: the RT (Respiratory Therapist) was checking the patient's ventilations and considering setting up an automated ventilator; another nurse was cutting his clothes; another was getting ready to start a second IV; another was setting up the whole blood administration set; another was charting and recording everything. It was like a swarm of bees working to save this man's life. Shortly after a pulse check, they announced that the man was in cardiac arrest and a staff member was instructed to begin CPR. As I looked on, another two ER doctors entered and there were other staff who looked on as various interventions were done.

I began feeling an adrenaline dump and began moving the cot out of the trauma room. I went back to the car to begin recording times and complete my PCR (Patient Care Record), as I did not have time during the call. Everything had to be recorded in chronological order. I obtained times off of our CAD and noted that our on-scene time was only five minutes from the time we pulled up to the time that we were en route to the hospital. This was an excellent departure time, with limited time on scene; in a case like this, minutes counted, and any delays reaching a trauma room could mean this man's life. Paul the ALS Paramedic came over and we talked briefly about the call. He said he was going to write inside where it was cooler. I finished recording my times and headed inside also, as the sun was warming the inside cab of the Ambulance and making it uncomfortable.

Just as I was about to enter the ER, another ambulance pulled up with its lights flashing and backed into the bay beside us. It was the second stabbing victim, picked up one block from where our patient was stabbed. They unloaded, and I found out it was a non-life-threatening stab to the right deltoid. I wondered if it was the same person who stabbed our patient.

After entering the hospital, I proceeded to the trauma room to see how the man was making out. To my surprise, they has cut open his chest, just below the xyphoid process, from his left armpit to his right. One doctor had her hand inside his chest and was performing manual cardiac massage, while another was attempting to find and clamp off the bleeding artery. A huge gush of blood (approximately a litre) was spilling out the right side of his chest onto the trauma bed, pooling in a containment barrier. The second doctor was working feverishly to find the bleeding artery and stop it. I looked at the two bags of whole blood hanging and being infused. I thought 'They can't get the blood in fast enough from what is flowing out.' I watched for a few minutes with the rest of the audience; there must have been seventeen people surrounding the patient including all the staff working to keep him alive. They then were going to cut his sternum. A staff member arrived with a huge shear; it looked like something used to trim branches on a tree and had handles almost two feet long. The staff member began to cut into the bone until the doctor doing cardiac massage instructed her to stop. They had another plan. A cardiac and vascular surgeon arrived to take over the management of the bleeding artery.

I finally excited the trauma room and walked over to the counter where Paul was writing his PCR. I walked up and said: "Paul, you should go back inside and check that out. They have his entire chest cut open. Never seen that in the ER before."

Paul replied: "Naw, I actually don't like to see that. I can do a call fine, but watching that from a distance does not sit well with me so I'll pass." He gave me a small smile. I looked at him with I'm sure what was a surprised look. I replied: "Oh...OK."

I finished my paperwork and exited the ER. My partner, Tim, was talking to another paramedic. I said: "Hey, I am going to walk down to Starbucks to grab a coffee before we clear." Tim replied: "Sure, I'm just getting caught u; we used to work together."

I enjoyed the short walk a few blocks away to the Starbucks as my adrenaline rush began leaving my body. After getting back, we cleaned up the back of our Ambulance, re-stocking and replacing items as required.

As we left the hospital, Tim and I talked about the call. As we crossed a bridge back to our area, we heard the CAD blip and a message appeared. It was our dispatcher asking us if we were OK or needed some time before we cleared for our next call. Tim and I talked a minute and we were both OK to clear. We cleared and were promptly given a three-car MVA on another bridge over twenty minutes away.

Partner du jour

My regular partner was on vacation for the block so an irreg Paramedic was assigned to work with me for the block. We had worked together in the past and it had been a good experience, so I was looking forward to the block. He was an East Indian guy (Jag) with a rather unique personality; we had always had rather unique conversations during our shifts. It was my second day back and it was my normal attend day. We had already started with a busy block on the previous day.

It was 1742 and we were in quarters when the hotline rang. We had been assigned cross-coverage to an area that was a twenty-minute drive from us. We were not looking forward to it as we were due to be off shift at 1830 and were not interested in doing any late calls. After working twelve hours, I was normally done for the day; the OT was not worth it.

Jag headed out and we made our way to the cross-coverage location rather slowly, hoping to be cancelled before we got there. Just then, the CAD sounded: "Blip...blip...blip." I spun the CAD toward me a looked at the screen:

- Response: Code 3
- Call Source: Person at scene
- Type: OD
- Units: 75A3
- Remarks: Possible narcotic drug overdose
- FD responding

Jag lit it up and activated the siren, while I looked at the integrated map to see our best access to the location. It was a residence so there were no elevators to worry about. We were not close to the call, so it took us approximately twelve minutes, Code 3 to arrive. When we pulled up, Fire was on scene. It was a new subdivision in a very upscale area — not what we normally would have expected from a narcotic OD.

We exited, and I said: "If you can just grab the O2 that would be great" Jag replied: "Sure thing."

I grabbed the kit and unconscious arrest bag that contained the AED, and suction. We headed in together. As we entered, a man in his early 20s greeted us: "It's my brother. He is not responding, and I think he OD."

I said: "Does he normally do drugs?"

The man replied: "Yeah, he has been dealing with a heroin addiction for some time now."

As we entered the living room of the well-kept home, we saw a Caucasian man lying supine on the hard wood floor. The two firefighters had just arrived; they were measuring an OPA and had a BVM ready to ventilate the man. I reached toward his wrists and felt for a radial pulse. His pulse was present, weak, and rapid. I observed his breathing rate and he was breathing at a rate of eight breaths per minute. I scanned his body and there were no pools of blood, and no obvious deformities. I opened the kit and placed the pulse oximeter on his finger. The display light up and read 'Pulse rate of 135 Spo2 78%.' I looked at his face: his lips were cyanotic and his skin pale. When I opened his eye lids, his pupils were pinned at 2mm each, and non-reactive.

I looked at the firefighters and said: "If you guys can bag him I will check his sugar." Jag was speaking with the brother, getting details on how he was found, etc. I popped open the kit, grabbed the glucometer kit, poked the patient's finger, and obtained a blood sample; the reading was 5.7mmol. Anything above 4mmol was considered normal, so I now ruled out a diabetic emergency. I looked over at the Spo2 monitor and it now read 98%.

I said: "Great job bagging him."

I grabbed an NPA airway, picked a French 34, lubed it, and had the firefighters stop bagging him for a minute. I choose the left nostril and, with a few small twists, inserted the six-inch rubber airway into his nose until it stopped at his nostril. The firefighters already had an OPA inserted but I wanted an additional airway, and the NPAs were more effective in many ways than the OPAs. Also, when patients are decreased GCS but still have a gag reflex, they will often accept an NPA but not an OPA. The firefighters continued bagging the patient.

I said: "Jag, I am going to draw up the Narcan."

Jag replied: "OK...so the brother here said he found his brother down on the floor, had not seen him for a few hours, so unknown how long he has been down. He is also on house arrest and has an ankle bracelet on."

I stopped what I was doing, looked down at his ankles, and pulled up his jeans a bit, exposing an ankle bracelet on his right leg.

I returned to the kit, pulled out the med box, selected an ampule of 1cc 0.4mg Narcan, and flicked it with my right index finger as I held it with my left thumb and forefinger; this was to move the medication from the top part of the ampule back into the main part before I drew it up. I selected a 3cc 1.5-inch IM needle and drew up the medication. I capped the needle until I was ready to administer it. I looked over and the firefighters were ventilating the patient adequately, while my partner had obtained a BP 136/78. I selected the patient's left should deltoid, inserted the needle like a dart, and withdrew to check for blood in case I entered a vein. I then administered the Narcan, withdrew the needle, and pushed the button at the back of the syringe to retract the needle inside the syringe for safety. Now it was time to wait a few minutes. Normally, Narcan will begin having an effect in a few minutes, even with an IM administration.

After waiting three minutes with no change in the patient's mental status, I considered that he might have taken Fentanyl and he might require more Narcan. I said to Jag: "I'm going to give him another 0.4mg Narcan...see if that wakes him up." I drew up a second syringe of Narcan and administered it into his arm. We waited another three to four minutes with still no response.

Then, the patient suddenly began to vomit. Luckily, the firefighters were on it and quickly rolled the man onto his right side, as copious amounts of vomit began to pour out of his mouth onto the hardwood floor. I grabbed the portable electric suction and began to suction his mouth as he lay on his side.

Jag said: "Hey, think we should get going on this guy. I am going to grab the clam."

I replied: "OK, I was hoping he would wake up before we move him but looks like that might not be happening." Jag left for the equipment as the patient continued to vomit, spewing more vomit on the floor as the firefighters moved away so as not to contaminate themselves as they continued to hold him on his side. It was times like this that I was glad to be the Paramedic and able to stand back rather than be beside the patient while they are vomiting. I'm sure at this point the firefighters were thinking 'This is not what the fire fighter poster said.'

By the time Jag returned with the clam shell, the man had stopped his vomiting for the time being. Jag said: "Let's move him away from the vomit so we can get the clam under him."

I replied: "Sounds good. Think he will vomit again...was hoping he would stop before we loaded him, so we don't have to deal with an airway issue."

Jag said: "Yeah, I hear you, but thinking we should begin packaging regardless." I knew Jag was right, but things get complicated with packaging a patient lateral on a clam, especially when, during a move, the patient begins to vomit again. In these cases, we have to stop the Ambulance to suction and deal with the airway; we had done this many times in the past.

We split the clam in two parts and slid it underneath his body as he was supported on his left side. After, we secured the straps snugly to ensure he did not slide back onto his back.

Jag said: "I have the cot outside ready to go."

I replied: "Perfect, let's go before he vomits again."

We lifted him and began the move. When we loaded him into the Amb, I climbed in after him. I re-checked his airway; as I did, he vomited again — luckily a smaller amount than before. I suctioned his airway as he was on his side, so there was no aspiration. Jag closed the doors. Shortly afterwards he said: "Are you ready to roll Code 3 or Routine?"

I replied: "Yes, we had better make it Code 3, and can you hand me the cell?

Jag replied, "Sure," and handed me the cell through the bulk-head window.

As we headed out Jag activated the siren. I began getting IV supplies ready, applied a tourniquet and began looking for an appropriate vein; I wanted one where I could use an 18G catheter. I found one, prepped the site, and laid out everything nearby: Tegaderm, gauze, tape, interlock connector, and 1000cc bag of NaCl with tubing primed. I looked out the front window to see when we might approach a light; depending on how rough the road was, I might attempt a start on the roll, but if I thought we would hit a patch of rough road, I planned to have my partner pull over. The last thing I needed was to just have begun insertion then be tossed around, missing the vein and increasing the possibility of a needle stick injury.

I called out to Jag: "Hey, about to start a line. Can you pull over for a minute?"

Jag replied: "Sure, I can stop in a few secs."

As the Amb slowed to a stop, I was ready. As soon as it was still, I inserted an 18G catheter. It went in smoothly. I applied the tegaderm, taped it in place, and began adjusting the flow control regulator...it was patent and flowing well. I called out: "OK, thanks. We can carry on."

I then opened the older style flip cell phone. It was funny that we still used them when everyone was using high tech touchscreen Android and iPhones; nonetheless, these served our purpose because they had the numbers we needed programmed in and they lasted days on a single charge. I selected 'EPOS' and hit 'Send.' It began dialing and after a few rings I heard a voice: "Doctor Newton."

I said: "Hi Doctor, this is Luciano with BC Ambulance. I'm a PCP. I have a thirty-seven-year-old Caucasian male who is suspected of an opiate overdose at home. When we arrived his O2 sats were 78% on room air, breathing at a rate of 8 and shallow. His pupils were pinned and non-responsive. His pulse was tacky at 135 and strong at the radials, B/P 136/78. There was no obvious trauma and his brother who called us says he has a history of heroin use. I have given two 0.4mg Narcan IM with 3-4 minutes between with no change in mental status. His

Glucose is 5.7. He did vomit a large amount after the second injection. I have an 18G IV infusing and I am currently considering more Narcan but would like a consult on options before I give any more. He is on a cannula now and his sats are now 97%."

Doctor Newton replied: "Well, sounds like you have covered all the bases at this point. How far are you from the hospital?"

"About eight minutes."

Doctor Newton replied: "Well, given you will be there shortly, I would hold off on more Narcan. There is a risk of putting him into a rapid detox and it could exacerbate the problem with the possibility of seizures."

I said: "OK, thanks, appreciate that. I was not sure if more Narcan would benefit him. He is maintaining his sats now."

Doctor Newton replied: "Sure, no problem. Do you have the response number handy?"

I said: "Yes, it's 345987."

Doctor Newton replied: "Thanks. If you need anything else just call me back."

I said: "Sure, will do. Appreciate it." I hung up the cell.

We arrived at the hospital shortly afterward and brought the patient into the ER. I gave the hand-over report and he was given a bed shortly afterward. After we finished up, we were looking forward to getting off work; it was almost an hour of OT at this point.

On duty or off?

We were sitting at our station — a rare occurrence. I even had my feet up on the recliner. There was one other crew in the station, but we were 'up car.' (When multiple cars are at the station, the first one back is the next one out on the next call and this continues down the line. Sometimes we are 'quadruple down,' but that does not last very long as, sometimes, when the hotline rings, there will be multiple calls all at once and the station clears quickly.)

The hotline rang. It was a red phone with a very distinctive loud ring to it. It is a direct line to the dispatcher so that, when you pick it up, it auto-dials the dispatcher. There is no keypad on the phone. I answered the phone: "Alpha 3."

Dispatch: "I have a Code 3 on the CAD, unconscious, still coming in."

I replied: "OK, we are on it." I hung up the phone and my partner said: "What do we have?"

"Code 3, unconscious."

We both headed out to the bay, opened the doors and climbed in. I spun the CAD toward me and read the call:

- Location: Mall – North entrance
- Response: Code 3
- Type: Unconscious/ Cardiac arrest suspected
- Call source: Person on scene
- Units: 75A3, 75A1
- Remarks:
  - 10:02 Male, age unknown, breathing rate unknown
  - 10:03 Male, unconscious, age unknown.
  - 10:04 Fire dept. responding
  - 10:05 Bystanders CPR in progress – Cardiac arrest suspected/confirmed.

I said: "It looks like an arrest at the mall. We are only six minutes away."

Jag said, "Let's do it," spun the CAD toward him, looked at the call, and began writing on his clip board.

The radio squawked: "75A3 you have 75A1 fifteen minutes away."

I grabbed the mike and said: "75A3, 10-4."

I pulled out of the bay and, once we cleared the doors, activated the emergency lights; when we approached a nearby intersection, I turned on the siren. Traffic stopped after a couple of cars passed by. I knew our time to the call counted, so I pushed it and drove faster than I often do on many of our Code 3 calls, alternating the siren tones from hyper-help to hi/low to phaser. I used the airhorn especially at intersections to get drivers' attention in their virtually soundproof vehicles.

The CAD blipped again, and Jag read out the screen. "It says to take the back entrance near the Tim Hortons."

I replied: "OK, I know the one. Does it say if anyone is going to meet us at the entrance and guide us to the scene?"

Jag replied: "No."

I grabbed the mike and said: "75A3."

Dispatch: "75A3."

I said: "Is anyone meeting us at the door to guide us in?"

Dispatch: "75A3, security said they would meet you at the entrance."

I said: "10-4."

I pulled up to the entrance quickly, scaring a few people standing near the entrance. As I got out, I could smell the brakes due to the hard driving on the way to the call. Jag exited. I went to the back, pulled out the cot, placed the O2 tank on it, and wheeled it around the side toward the entrance to the mall. Jag had grabbed the kit and the resuscitation kit (AED and suction). He placed it on the cot as I was pushing it onto the mall. We looked around but there was no security.

I said: "Great, no security. They said near the Starbucks, didn't they?"

Jag replied: "Yeah, I know where it is…just up there to the left."

We quickly wheeled our cot loaded with equipment through the mall. People shopping stared at us as we proceeded. Finally, a security guard approached us from the direction we were heading. As he got within talking distance I said: "Hey, I thought there was going to be someone to meet us at the door?"

The guard said: "Yes, we were all tied up dealing with this." I looked at him a bit stunned and glanced back at Jag who also had one of those eye rolling looks on his face. I replied: "Well maybe, but until we get there, treatment is limited."

Jag said: "So what is happening?"

The guard said: "We are doing CPR on him."

As we rolled around past the Starbucks kiosk, we could see people around a man lying on the floor. There was a security guard performing chest compressions, while other security were standing nearby keeping people away. As we pulled up I noticed an AED connected to the man's chest. There were no signs of trauma and I noticed he was a Caucasian man in his late 20s or early 30s. He was a heavyset man weighing over 190lbs. They had an O2 mask on his face and his colour was pale but not cyanotic, as I would have expected from someone in cardiac arrest.

Jag said: "Luc can you go manage the airway?"

I replied: "Sure."

I grabbed the kit, placed it on the ground nearby and pulled out the BVM and OPA airways. Just then, the AED sounded: "Check for sign of life." The security guard doing compressions had moved off the chest and a woman not in uniform was landmarked for compressions. The AED sounded: "Continue CPR." The woman began compressing the patient's chest as I moved in near his head and felt for a carotid pulse; there was a strong carotid pulse.

I yelled out: "He has a pulse. Stop CPR."

The woman on the chest continued compressing. I said again: "Stop CPR. He has a pulse." I pushed on her arms to move her off his chest, as she was in the moment and focused on what she was doing. She finally paused and looked at me.

I said: "He has a strong pulse; you can get off his chest." She moved off his chest as I reached for his radial pulse: it was also present. That confirmed his BP was reasonable and within a closer to normal range, though he was still unconscious. The woman identified herself as a nurse.

Jag was busy getting a history, so I grabbed the kit, opened it, and placed the pulse ox on the patient's finger; it read '95% SPO2 pulse rate of 88.' I looked through the OPA bag, as the yellow airway in place seemed to be too small based on the size of the man's jaw. I considered replacing it with a red airway or adding a NPA in addition to it. I had begun to vent the man with the BVM when the Fire Department arrived. One firefighter moved in to take over airway and bagging for me. We normally prefer the fire crews do that for us so that we can manage the call, initiate IVs, give medications, and plan to transport the patient.

The ALS crew arrived, and Jag gave the report. We had to load the man onto the cot with the clam shell as he remained unconscious. There was some presumption that he had had a seizure. The ALS crew transported, and I drove them in as we needed both in the back to manage the patient.

No DNR?

We were working my usual area on our way to a routine call for a MVA about 1km from our location. We were in heavy afternoon traffic on a cold, December day. There was lots of ice on the side roads and 10cm snow on areas that were not cleared. We had snow early this year, only a few days into December. My partner was driving, and it was my second day of vacation recall on this ambulance with him. Due to being so short-staffed, we could work non-stop, seven days a week. Getting called in for vacation recall was double time, so most of us were willing to pick up a few shifts.

Just then, the CAD sounded: "Blip...blip...blip." Then the radio sounded: "34B1 cancel your last. I have a Code 3 on your CAD. ALS not available."

I spun the CAD toward me and read the call out loud: "It's Cardiac arrest...looks like we are only a few blocks away. If you spin around and go back down to 45th Ave, it is only a few blocks from there."

My partner, James, began looking for a place to turn around, but traffic was heavy. He managed to find a place to turn around, navigating through the annoying centre medians. They seem to put them up everywhere for traffic separation, but it makes responding to emergency calls a nightmare. Seconds count in a cardiac arrest; had there been no traffic and an ability to turn around, we would have been there already.

James found a place to turn around, activated the emergency lights and siren, and began heading to the call.

I began reading the notes on the CAD: "90yo female..." I said: "Great, she is ninety years old...and sounds like no DNR. I don't want to do compressions on a ninety-year-old."

James replied: "Yeah, sucks, feeling the cartilage and bones cracking as you begin compressions, and why? At ninety she is in arrest because she is dying." James shook his head side to side as he spoke.

I began writing on my PCR and thinking of the call and what to expect. We never know — the patient could be in a bedroom, living room, kitchen, garage, or outside. There are so many variables and every call is unique.

We pulled up to a nice rancher-style residence that was well-kept in a nice, clean neighbourhood. I grabbed the jump kit and recess kit (AED, Suction) and James grabbed the O2 from the back. I headed in first to the open front door. I entered a very tidy living room and an elderly woman was on the floor; above her was a woman in her sixties doing what I believe she thought was chest compressions. As I moved closer, I realized she was actually going through the motions but not actually compressing the chest, bending her elbows rather than pressing the chest down. I moved toward the head of the woman on the floor; she was old, had cyanotic lips, and was ashen pale.

I said: "Stop, please move aside," but the woman continued. I repeated myself: "Stop, I need to assess this woman." The woman stopped and frantically looked at me. She said: "This is my mom."

I checked the patient's carotid pulse as I said, "Did you see her collapse?" Just then, James entered the room. The daughter replied: "Yes, yes! She collapsed right in front of me."

I said: "OK, James, we have a witnessed arrest. Patient has no pulse." I moved and opened the kit, grabbing the BVM and airways.

James said: "I'll take care of the airway if you want to begin compressions and attach the AED."

I paused a moment as my brain processed this. I did not want to do compressions and was hoping James would have landmarked; it looked like I was the one. I exposed the chest to reveal a frail, boney chest. I opened the AED and attached the pads to the upper right and lower left chest. When I turned it on it sounded "Beep, beep, beep...Start CPR." I landmarked and began compressions. Just as I suspected, the cracks could be heard throughout the room. I cringed inside as I compressed at a rate of 100 per minute. After three compressions, the cracks stopped, and it became a mechanical action.

After two minutes of CPR, the AED sounded: "Press Analyze, and stand clear." I pressed the 'Analyze' button and the AED again sounded: "Stand clear, analyzing now." I looked up to make sure James was not touching the patient or the daughter. The AED sounded again: "No shock advised. Begin CPR."

As we began our second round of CPR, the Fire Crew arrived with three men. I said: "Can one of you get ready to take over? I am going to start a line." One of the firefighters positioned himself on the other side of the patient, waiting.

The Fire Captain said: "I'll find out the history."

James said: "And find out if there is a DNR. She was attempting CPR, so we assume no."

To the firefighter across from me I said: "OK, get ready to get in and continue compressions."

He replied: "I'm ready." I stopped and moved off the chest. The firefighter landmarked and began compressions immediately.

I said: "OK, you have about thirty seconds left before we have to analyze."

I pulled out the IV start kit and began prepping the right AC for an IV. I attempted a start, but the frail veins would not allow a start. A moment later, the Fire Captain walked in the room and said: "We have a DNR."

I said: "Is it for this woman? The daughter was attempting compressions when we walked in."

The Captain said, "Yes, matches the name," as he handed me the DNR document. I began reading the information; just then ALS walked in. I said out loud, "We have a DNR," and handed it to the ALS crew, but did not say 'Stop CPR' at this point; I had never had a DNR presented to me by the same family that had initiated CPR.

A moment after the ALS crew member read the document, he said: "Stop CPR." The firefighter stopped compressions and my partner backed away from the BVM.

I paused in thought as I absorbed this new information. We didn't want to start CPR when we walked in, and now to find a DNR after almost six minutes of CPR sucked. I cleaned up the equipment and cut the AED wires to leave in place for the coroner. We covered the woman with a blanket and I left to complete paperwork while my partner stayed with the family, advising them that the police were going to attend and why.

I returned to the Ambulance and began filling in my PCR. I looked at the woman's age and the CAD was wrong: She was ninety-six-years-old, not ninety. 'Great,' I thought, 'that is even worse!' My stomach went into a knot as I thought of the first few compressions and the cracking and feel of the chest collapsing; I had a shudder. I completed my PCR in detail as the police would want a copy for their report. After I was done, I headed back to the residence as James was walking out with the O2 bottle.

I said: "I will stay with the family if you like. My paperwork is done."

James said: "OK, I will re-stock the kits then."

I replied: "Great!"

I entered the residence and spoke with the daughter and her husband. I soon realized that she was in denial that her mother was dying. Even though the DNR had been signed a few months earlier, she could not consciously accept that her mother was going to die, so began CPR. After about twenty minutes I noticed a police car drive by and stop; I informed them I would go out and speak to the officer. I went out talked with the officer, handing him a copy of the PCR. I went back into the residence briefly to let the family know we were leaving and the officer would be right in to talk with them. I returned to the car and climbed in. James was listening to music and sending a text.

James said: "All done?"

I replied: "Yeah, sure would have been nice to know she had a DNR before we began resuscitation. Hate compressing on old people's chests when they are dying. Why can people not accept that people are going to die? She was ninety-six, not ninety!"

James began driving forward and said: "Yeah, I know. It sucks."

We continued on in silence, listening to the radio as we headed back to the station, which was only seven minutes from the location of the call. We were now into overtime and wanted to be done for the day, so we didn't clear the call on our CAD as we knew that if we did another would pop up on the screen.

Wear your seatbelt

We were a three-person crew on this day, as I had a student and was precepting. It was her second week and she was keen and excited (like most new students) to get some interesting calls. Interesting calls to a student are usually something traumatic or where the pressure is on to make critical decisions. Normally, the patient is very sick or injured and requires immediate intervention to preserve life until we are able to get them to a hospital. Paramedics are an odd group in that the more serious the call, the more we want to be involved with it. We never want anyone to die or suffer, but nonetheless find it an adrenaline rush to push our assessment and training to the limit to stabilize and keep people alive.

My partner was a part-timer out of post and was driving. We were having a normal, busy, non-stop day, dealing with syncope events, falls from standing, or general illness. We were currently on our way to a ninety-five-year-old woman who was unable to get up out of a chair. Her daughter was en route to open the door, as she was a key holder and did not want us to breach the door.

Suddenly, the dispatcher called us on the radio: "75A3."

My partner gabbed the mike: "75A3."

Dispatch: "75A3, cancel your last. Begin Code 3 to Highway Number 1 for a multi-car MVA. Will get back to you with exact location."

My partner replied: "10-4."

She activated the emergency lights and sirens, but we were already heading in the direction of the call. The traffic was busy as it was late afternoon and commuters were heading home from work.

The CAD blipped and displayed the following:

- Location: Hwy Westbound
- Response: Code 3
- Type: 29D05 (Traffic Accident – Pinned (trapped) victim – multiple pts)
- Call source: Person at scene
- Units: 75A3, 45B1, 55A1,55C1,280B1, 21P2, 34A2
- Remarks:
  - 1625:01 Chief Complaint: 1 UNCONS – ROLL OVER MVI, age unknown, gender unknown, breathing status unknown, consciousness unknown, multiple patients: 2
  - 1625:32 Fire responding
  - 1625:40 Duty supervisor paged
  - 1626:54 1 Pt trapped
  - 1626:56 Significant event
  - 1627:12 Auto launch Helo requested
  - 1629:39 Police notified
  - 1630:10 2 adults (1 u/c – 1 conscious) no children
  - 1631:05 Duplicate call received

As I looked at the details coming through the CAD, I read them out to my partner. I looked at where we were and gave some instructions on the best routing to the call location, based on local knowledge and traffic patterns. I called back to the student and said: "Well, looks like you get a trauma call today."

The student replied: "Yes, I sure will."

My partner was focused on driving and navigating through the moderately heavy traffic, often going against oncoming lanes to pass intersections with medians. The radio was going constantly, with the dispatcher assigning multiple cars to respond to the accident.

I grabbed the mic at one point at a critical turning intersection and said: "Break, 75A3, we would like to know if the accident is East or West of the overpass?"

Dispatch: "The scene is just past the overpass, westbound."

I replied: "10-4."

I noticed my partner was going to proceed through the intersection when we needed to turn left. I yelled at my partner: "Turn left!!"

She replied: "OK, was not sure as we were going to gain access farther up."

I said: "Yes, I know. That's why I called to clarify. The location was not clear. All good...we are in a good place for access."

As we crossed over the overpass to the highway, we looked down and traffic was at a standstill; we could see a fire truck approaching the underpass as well as a supervisor.

I shouted out again to my partner: "Turn right onto the ramp!!" She moved to the right, almost passing the on-ramp. I could see she was stressed and doing the best she could in all the confusion.

There was heavy, slow traffic on the ramp due to the accident just on the other side of it. My partner navigated her way through traffic, alternating the siren tones as we went. As we rounded the corner, we could see the supervisor SUV drive past slowly on the highway, with a fire truck right behind him.

We pulled up to the right side of the concrete blocks separating the onramp from the highway. As we rolled up we could see a white SUV flipped on the driver's side. Farther across the lanes was a full-sized pickup truck that had some front-end damage. I had already put my blue nitrile gloves on and grabbed my personal safety vest as I exited the door. Cars were still passing by the right side of our Ambulance as traffic proceeded to merge with the highway farther up. I shouted back to the student: "Make sure your safety vest is on and exit the rear of the car."

She replied: "Sure, will do."

I got out, grabbed the kit out of the side compartment, and headed around back toward the flipped SUV. I noticed a few people walking about and a man crouched down near the open sun-roof of the flipped vehicle. A man approached us and said: "There is a guy in that car" — he motioned toward the flipped SUV — "that is unconscious and trapped." He continued, "There is also two more people that were in the truck," and pointed toward the back of a full-sized SUV.

I replied: "OK, thanks."

I moved in toward the more serious of the injured, the man in the smaller SUV. A man in a safety vest was holding c-spine on the driver through the sun-roof. Two firefighters were at the vehicle side as I hopped over the three-foot high concrete dividers.

I spoke to the firefighters: "We might need the jaws to cut that roof off."

The one firefighter said: "Sure thing. Let us know what you need."

As I approached he said: "I just lost his pulse. He had a pulse thirty seconds ago."

My mind flashed with the situation: The patient was in an overturned SUV, and I was told he was trapped and unconscious. Now, I had just been informed that his pulse stopped. I could smell the strong odour of gasoline, and the road was wet with a combination of water from the radiator, fuel, and oil. I quickly moved in and reached inside the truck to feel for the man's carotid pulse. I waited for ten seconds and could feel nothing. I knew we could do nothing for him while he was inside the flipped truck. If the Fire Department would have to use the jaws to cut him out, he would not make it as it would take at least ten to fifteen minutes to set up the jaws and remove the roof to gain access. I looked at the man's face: it was lifeless and pale. His legs were still under the dash and I noticed he was not wearing a seatbelt. All the airbags in the vehicle had deployed.

I shouted out: "He has no pulse...we have to get him out!" I shouted to the man still holding c-spine: "Give me a hand pulling him out!"

I grabbed the top of his shoulders, and under his armpits, and the other man grabbed the other side. The patient was wearing a winter jacket and, as we began pulling, the unconscious man moved a bit toward the sunroof, but his jacket began to pull up from his torso. This man was dead weight; his legs were pinned under the dash and I had no idea if his legs were trapped.

I said: "Come on, we have to get him out. Keep pulling."

I tried to support his limp head as best as I could. We continued to pull on him as I heard paramedics' voices say: "Get the spine board"... "Place the monitor over there"..."We have to be ready when he comes out." In a few moments, with the combined effort of the other man and myself, we pulled the patient free of the vehicle. We continued to drag him away from the wet fuel and water, approximately twenty feet from the vehicle.

As soon as we stopped I shouted out: "Let's get his jacket off." I pulled from behind his jacket and it slipped off over his head with ease. He was placed back on the roadway in a supine position. I moved in to check his pulse again at the carotid for approximately ten seconds. I felt nothing. I shouted out: "No pulse."

Next, I exposed the chest and placed my left hand on his mid sternum, my right hand over the top. I began compressing hard and fast at a rate of 100 per minute. I looked over to the patient's head; one of the ALS paramedics that had arrived in the papa car inserted an OPA and began bagging him. I continued compressing the chest as someone else placed defibrillator pads on the chest.

I noticed my student and said: "You are going to be doing compressions." She moved to my side and I said: "Go over to the other side and get ready." She moved to the other side of the man. I said: "OK, I am going to move off the chest and you just continue compressions OK?" She replied: "Yes...OK."

I moved quickly from the chest and my student placed her hands on the chest and began compressing. I then moved back out of the way and stood up. I looked down at the man: CPR in progress, ALS intubating the man, monitor hooked up. I looked over the scene: there were police, paramedics and firefighters moving about. I heard someone say: "Someone said that there were kids in the car. Has the car been searched yet?"

I moved over to the SUV, looked inside the back window, and noticed two car seats: they were empty. I moved around to the sunroof and peered inside. I could see the car seats, but it was dark inside due to the tinted windows. There was a firefighter also looking inside the car. I climbed on the passenger side of the flipped SUV and peered inside the vehicle. The tinted windows continued to make it difficult. In addition, the curtain airbags were also obscuring our view inside. I then reached down to my duty belt, removed my rescue knife, and set the spring-operated window breaker.

I called out to the firefighter: "I'm going to break the window."

He replied: "That's a good idea."

I placed the retracted window breaker against the glass and flipped the lever on the side of my knife. As the spring-activated pin contacted the glass there was a 'pop' sound as the glass turned from clear to shattered. I began pushing the glass inward but was only wearing my nitrile gloves. The firefighter noticed and began clearing the glass away with his work gloves on. I then tried to stab into the still-inflated curtain airbag with my knife. My rescue knife was flat tipped for safety and would not puncture the tough airbag material. I then began cutting the attachment anchors that keep the airbag in position along the edge of the doorway. After cutting the curtain airbag away, I used my tactical light to illuminate the inside of the car. I could not see any children in the car. The firefighter was looking from another vantage point and could not see anyone either. I was satisfied and dismounted the vehicle.

I looked over the scene: ALS was working on the man I had help pull out; there were RCMP officers scattered all over the place, many interviewing people off to the side; other Paramedics were dealing with other patients, two of whom were placed on stretchers on clam shells. I noticed there was no stretcher set up for the man that was still in cardiac arrest, so I went back to our Ambulance, pulled out the stretcher, and removed the blankets and pillow. I pulled out the clam shell. As I turned, the cot had rolled away from the Amb onto the laneway as there was a slight incline. I took ten steps and retrieved the cot, moved it back beside the concrete barriers, and placed the clam, a collar, and head bed on it. I crossed over the concrete barriers and noticed a firefighter was holding the IV bag for the crews working the arrest.

I walked over and said: "I can hold that now if you like?"

The firefighter said: "OK."

As I held the IV, I looked back and noticed the traffic on the Eastbound lane was passing by slowly. I wondered if the people driving past could see us doing CPR on this man on the roadway. I turned toward the crews working on this man. I noticed the IV 250c bag I was holding was getting low. Seeing my partner nearby, I said: "Hey Stephanie, can you grab a 1000cc bag from the suction bag; this one is getting pretty low."

Stephanie replied: "Sure."

She looked through the Suction/Arrest kit and pulled out a 1000cc Nacl bag and walked over and handed it to me. I placed it near the kit on the roadway, anticipating the need for it soon.

The ALS were commenting on the man's condition and he had a PE. They began to insert large intrathoracic needles to decompress his chest. The first needle was placed over the left chest, mid clavicular line, just below the second rib. After insertion, blood oozed from the end of the needle. This indicated a hemothorax. If that side of the chest was full of blood, the outcome for this man was grim. I looked on as they inserted a second IV into the right side of the chest at same position as the left. This time no blood or air escaped. Due to the small size of the needles inserted (14G) there was little chance that doing so would cause a pneumothorax; in this case, the field assessment of a tension pneumothorax was not accurate. The needle decompression can dramatically change the outcome of a patient with a tension pneumothorax present.

As I stood there, another paramedic I knew walked over to me. He said: "Hey Luch how are you doing?" He had a look of concern on his face. He was a very seasoned paramedic and this scene was not something he had not seen before either. I felt he was just checking up on me.

I replied: "I'm OK, thanks Bob."

He said: "Think this guy is going to make it?"

I replied: "It's not looking good. Think they are going to call it soon."

Bob walked away, and I stood there as the ALS paramedic in charge of the arrest stood up, walked over to me with the cell phone in his hand, and said: "I'm calling this. He has sustained too much trauma."

They were still doing CPR on him the paramedic made the call. I stood there just thinking about the crash scene. I was thinking that this man had a family and they were never going to talk to him again. His kids would never know their father. He would never see his kids grow up. Life can be taken so quickly. The man in the other full-sized truck had been heading Eastbound on Highway #1, crossed over the median, and crashed head-on into this man's van. This could have happened to anyone, and the timing of this event always seemed so odd. Had he been five seconds sooner, he would have been missed; but then, who knows — someone else might have been involved in the collision.

The ALS paramedic instructed the crew working on the man to stop resuscitation efforts. The person at the head stopped bagging and the person on the chest doing compressions stopped compressing. That was it. I looked down at the lifeless body lying on the roadway, the smell of gasoline and oil in the air. I could hear the sound of vehicles driving past. The flashing emergency lights from all the vehicles flickered.

I closed off the IV flow chamber, then moved around the man's body and tied off the IV tubing near the IO insertion site at his right tibia. Other paramedics were adjusting other equipment before we covered him with a blanket. It was required to keep IVs inserted and ET tubes in place for the coroner to see when he or she arrived.

I grabbed a blanket, and with a firefighter placed it over the man's body, completely covering him from head to toe.

I headed back to the stretcher that was still on the other side of the concrete barrier. My partner and I made up the cot and loaded it back into our Ambulance. The ALS paramedic came up to me and said: "The police will want your completed paperwork before you leave the scene."

I replied: "OK."

My partner, who had earlier had the vehicle insurance papers in her hand, made me wonder if we had confirmed his name and identity.

I said to her: "Hey, you had his insurance papers; do you still have them? I want his name for the PCR."

She replied: "I gave the insurance and his wallet to one of the police officers." She looked around to see if she could identify the officer. I looked around as well and the scene was littered with police. I would estimate there were at least 10 officers on scene. Despite asking a few of the police, we were unable to get the wallet and insurance papers back, so I headed back to our car to complete the paperwork.

I climbed into the cab of the Ambulance and began writing all the details of the call. The radio was blasting from other calls, so I turned the radio down to low. I turned on the FM radio and picked a music station to listen to while I reflected on the call. I looked up; there was still another ambulance on scene and numerous police milling about. While I was writing, my partner and student got in the Ambulance at one point, and we discussed points of the call. I realized that talking about the call was our way of defusing, but I was not getting my paperwork done.

The ALS paramedic came to the window and said: "I have my paperwork completed so don't think they will need yours as well. You guys can try to make it back to the station before getting another call."

I replied: "Thanks, OK. I am almost done. I will give it to them before we leave. I will be calling Dispatch as I umm…have some blood on my uniform and need a uniform change." I looked over at my partner as I spoke. She nodded and smiled.

The ALS paramedic said, "Yeah, I hate when that happens," smiling.

I completed our paperwork and brought it over to the RCMP officer who was working the file. As I walked back to the Ambulance I looked over at the blanket covering the man lying on the roadway. The police were investigating the accident, but there was nobody near the man's body. It was surreal as everyone detached and continued doing their job; this man was now dead and there was nothing else anyone could do. I called Dispatch and booked us out of service for uniform change.

The time was almost 1800hrs and we were off at 1830hrs. It would take us eighteen minutes to get back to the station from where we were anyway. As we drove, I looked down at my neon/green paramedic vest and noticed blood splatters on the bottom portion. It was only a small amount, but I did have the man's blood on my clothing as it turned out.

When we got back to the station we re-stocked as needed. Our Ambulance was out of service for the evening as they didn't have the staff to bring the car up in service. I scanned my paperwork and signed off my student's preceptor book. I decided to eat dinner and not rush home as there would be lots of traffic due to the highway being closed from the accident.

On my drive home, I kept visualizing the man's face in the overturned car, grabbing him with the other man and pulling him onto the roadway and starting CPR. I visualized the child seats in the back of the car and felt a rush of sadness that there was a family waiting for him that would never see him again. I felt a need to call my ex-wife and speak to my kids. I wanted to hear their voices to know I was thinking of them and how important they are to me; I only got voicemail. I tried to call my mom as I wanted to talk to someone; no answer. I even called an ex-girlfriend I stayed in touch with and it went to voicemail. The impact of this man's sudden death hit home with me this day. I realized that that could happen to me or anyone else in a moment. I wanted to connect with someone by voice that I had a connection with. I felt alone as the repeated visions of the man in the car, his face, the car seats, and him laying covered on the highway flashed in my mind. These visions continued for a couple of days then went away.

I had still been in treatment with my psychologist for my PTSD and asked her about it. I was told that it was a normal way of dealing with the event. I told her I normally don't ever have visions after calls and was concerned. She told me it was normal, especially since the visions only lasted a few days and disappeared. I felt relieved.

Trapped in an elevator

I was working my regular car with my regular partner. I had a student today and we had just left a major hospital from doing a transfer when the radio squawked:

Dispatch: "75A3."

My partner replied: "75A3."

Dispatch: "75A3, call coming in. Need you to turn back to the hospital. We have a man trapped in the elevator, cardiac history, Fire Department en route."

My partner: "10-4." He turned to me with one of those faces of disbelief. "They are sending an ambulance to a hospital for a man trapped in an elevator with a cardiac history?" He began laughing at this point.

I said: "That is nuts! Why are we responding inside a hospital for a man with a cardiac condition? Firstly, there is nothing we can do until we get to him, so we will be standing by with the Fire Department until they can get him out. Secondly, why can't they just bring him to the ER and have the nurses assess him? Talk about a waste of resources...wow!"

Just then the CAD sparked up: "Blip...blip...blip." I spun the screen and it read:

- Location: Trauma hospital
- Response: Code 3
- Type: Cardiac history, unknown
- Call source: Person on scene
- Units: 75A3
- Remarks:
  - Man trapped in Elevator, status unknown, cardiac history.
  - Fire responding

My partner spun the car around as we talked about the call. We were only a few blocks away from the hospital when the dispatcher called us again on the radio.

Dispatch: "75A3."

My partner: "75A3."

Dispatch: "75A3 you can cancel for a closer car."

My partner: "10-4."

He hung up the mic and, laughing, said: "What...did they find another crew in the hospital that could do the call?" I replied: "Yeah, or perhaps they realized that it is ludicrous to send an ambulance to a hospital for a man with a cardiac condition. Geez, really?"

We laughed about this call for a bit until the CAD blipped again; off we went to another call.

The Train

I was working de-paired on an Advanced Life Support ambulance during a night shift. We had a steady night so far with nothing very dramatic going on — a few SOB patients, but not critical. We made it back to the station and I took the opportunity to stretch out on one of the recliners and cover myself with a nice, soft fleece blanket, hoping to get a few minutes sleep before the next call.

I was asleep when that annoying sound awoke me: the hotline phone. I struggled to get up and answer it. The dispatcher told me we had a call. I headed out to the bay, listening for the movement of my partner in the crew bedroom to make sure he was awake. I entered the cab and looked at the notes on the CAD:

- Location: Train tracks
- Response: Code 3
- Type: Pedestrian struck (Major Trauma)
- Call source: Person on scene
- Units; 39A1, 65A2, 80

- Remarks:
  - Person possible hit by train, on tracks.
  - Train stopped
  - Fire Responding
  - Tracks have been deemed safe

As Adrian climbed into the cab I said: "Well, you wanted an exciting call...you just got one!"

He replied: "Yeah, no kidding?"

I pulled the car out of the bay and waited for the door to close as Adrian looked at the notes on the CAD and location of the call.

I said: "Is it just over the bridge?"

Adrian said: "Yeah, notes coming in now. I will call them to confirm the location."

I activated all the emergency lights and proceeded down the road. It was early morning around 5:00am, so morning traffic was just beginning to increase. As I approached the first intersection I turned on the siren. We were only six minutes from this call so not far at all. When we took the exit, we were given notes on how to get to the train crossing. On arrival, another BLS unit was on scene, as well as police and Fire Department.

I could see the train light down the tracks; it was probably 800 metres away and not at all close to the crossing we were at. We were still getting confirmation that the tracks were safe and the parallel tracks were shut down, as the West Coast Express travelled along the parallel tracks at that time of day.

I rolled down the window and the other paramedic from the BLS unit approached. Carl said: "Hey guys, so we are just getting confirmation that the tracks are shut down. I am trying to verify the best access as we may have a location closer to the train than from here."

Adrian said: "Sounds good, Carl. Let us know and we will follow you in."

I spun the Amb around and positioned us so we could follow the BLS unit in once they determined the best access and tracks shut down.

A few moments later, Carl called out to us: "OK, follow us. We are going down toward the train. I think I know where they are so we can access the patient easier."

I replied: "OK, sounds good."

They pulled out and we followed them with all our emergency lights flashing, making various turns as we did. Carl was a local and knew the area. He was also a part-time firefighter, so he was the best resource to determine the best access to the train and the patient.

We drove into an empty, dirt lot at the end of a road. I turned the Ambulance and positioned it for rapid exit if we had to load the patient and leave quickly. The other BLS crew got out and Adrian and I followed. We proceeded through some trees and uneven ground for about twenty-five feet then arrived at a four-foot-high fence.

I said: "Shouldn't we be bringing some equipment?"

Adrian replied: "We are just going to check this out."

Carl was already over the fence and I heard him say: "It's a confirmed Code 4." There was a man from the train talking with him. Adrian and I climbed over the fence; I was careful not to tear the crotch of my pants on the top of the chain-link fence. After getting over, we navigated through some brush and soft ground. My tactical light came in very handy to see the ground at this point. We came to a ditch approximately three feet across with soft ground.

Adrian said: "Can you shine your light on the ditch?"

I instinctively shone my light on the water and banks of the ditch. Adrian jumped over and I followed. Where Carl had guided us to park was literally right on top of where the person was hit by the train. I looked down to the distance and could see three flashlights and the silhouette of three bodies walking toward us from the crossing we had driven from.

Carl was about one hundred feet away shining his flashlight under the train, I could hear him saying: "Oh, yeah, definitely a Code 4."

Adrian and I walked over, and I shone my flashlight under the centre of a tanker car. It was a grisly and disturbing sight. I could see crumpled clothing; a small white breast was exposed, confirming in my mind a young female. Her body was bisected in the middle, and her intestines were hanging out. Her body was folded in half and her arms had been dismembered. Her head was visible, but her face was facing the other direction. I was glad about this, as when you see a dead person's face it changes how you process the event.

I said: "Wow, yeah, I would say a Code 4."

Carl said, "Unless you want to put the monitor on to make sure," as he chuckled.

Adrian replied, "Yeah, I don't think that will be necessary," in a sarcastic tone.

I said: "Hey, if you want the monitor on her, you can go back to the car and get it." I looked over at him with a grin.

We were all using dark humour as this wasn't anything to make jokes about. When we walked back over to the man with the train we found out he was the conductor. He said: "She just ran out in front of the train. There was nothing we could do to stop."

Carl said: "Sounds like a suicide."

After Adrian got some of the details he needed for his paperwork, we got a call from Dispatch on our portable radio.

Dispatch: "39A1, are you going to be tied up there? I have a Code 3 chest pain."

Adrian replied: "10-4."

Dispatch: "I will put it on your CAD."

The three silhouettes and flashlights arrived; it was the RCMP. I began to make my way back toward the ditch. Adrian was standing by the edge as we looked at the ditch.

I said: "Are you going to cross?"

Adrian replied with a laugh: "All yours buddy."

I had also been thinking what he had said. The ditch looked like it was farther across and a slip would mean landing in knee deep water. Neither of us really wanted to make the jump. I said: "OK, no problem." I had to sound confident as I leaped across the ditch and landed on the soft soil on the other side. Momentum was key as the other side of the ditch was sloped. Adrian followed after me and crossed without incident as well. We navigated back to the fence and vaulted it without catching any clothing in the process.

After getting back to the Ambulance I looked at the CAD, acknowledged the call, and read the notes. Adrian climbed in and I began to drive to the new call in a nearby town.

As I drove I thought of the visual image of the young woman with her guts hanging out. She looked in her early twenties, with fine features and a slim build. I thought about what had happened in her world that she would feel so desperate that she had to commit suicide.

Adrian tuned into the radio as we knew the commuter train that would normally pass on the parallel tracks would be shut down as part of the police investigation. The report on 1130 News Radio was already broadcasting that shuttle buses were being put into place to adjust for this sudden event that would now disrupt hundreds of people.

The Onion

It was a normal day at the station; I was sitting at the computer area when the hotline rang. I was next to the phone, so I picked it up and answered with my call sign: "32 Alpha 3."

The dispatcher voice said: "You are going to love this call."

I replied: "Oh, why is that? What have you got for us?"

The dispatcher said: "A guy's eyes are watering and burning from cutting an onion."

There was pause until I replied: "You are joking right?"

The dispatcher, now chuckling, said: "No, I'm not. I will throw it on your CAD."

I replied: "Perfect, I can't wait," laughing now.

I hung up the phone and my partner (Doug) who was standing nearby smiling, looked over at me and said: "What do we have that is so funny?"

I replied: "You won't believe this – you literally won't believe it. A guy called 911 because his eyes are burning from cutting an onion."

Doug said: "Seriously?"

I replied: "I know, right! I thought the dispatcher was just joking." I was laughing now.

"Well, let's go check this guy out" said Doug, smiling and laughing.

We walked out to the bay. Once we entered the car, we looked at the CAD, which read:

- Location: 2345 Orion street
- Response: Code 2
- Type: 16A1 eye problems/injuries – moderate eye injuries
- Call source: Person on scene
- Units: 32A3
- Remarks:
  - 18:42 Chief complaint, cutting onions, vision problems, seeing streaks 25-year-old male, conscious breathing.
  - 18:43 Caller I now away from the offending onion, has flushed his eyes, is still having vison problems.

After looking at the CAD I started laughing again and said: "The caller is away from the offending onion?"

Doug looked at the screen, smiling now and replied: "Well, that's a good thing; we don't want to be near any offending onions."

I was driving this evening, so I headed toward the call, which was only about 12 minutes away routine. I was pushing it a bit, as I wanted to get to this call, and I was still in disbelief that a 25-year-old called 911 for watering eyes from cutting an onion. As I drove I said: "We have to make it to this call. I want to meet this guy...what an idiot."

Laughing, Doug replied: "Maybe he has an onion allergy...this could be serious."

When we were a few blocks away I hit the 'arrive' button on the CAD so we could not be cancelled for another call. We pulled up to a multilevel home in a very nice neighborhood. I parked to the rear of the home. Before we exited, Doug said: "I want to take this guy to the hospital"

I replied: "What? Really? Why?"

Doug said: "Because nobody will believe us."

"Good point," I replied, laughing now.

Doug grabbed the jump bag and we headed up the stairs to the door. Doug knocked on the door and, after a few moments, the door opened. A young East Indian man in his 20s answered the door. He said: "Oh, I was going to call and cancel you guys."

Doug replied with a straight face: "Well, sir, we are here now and since you were concerned enough to call us we should check you out."

I also replied: "Yes, we should do a thorough medical assessment."

The man said: "Oh, ok, sure I guess."

He let us into the home. It was a very well kept, modern home, well decorated with high-end furnishings. A young boy, approximately 10-years-old, was also inside when we entered.

Doug said: "So, sir, is there someplace we can sit down and talk?"

The patient replied: "Sure, just over here." He motioned to the living room area where there were two couches and a chair. They moved into the room and sat on opposite couches as Doug began his assessment. Doug said: "So, can you tell me what happened?"

The patient said: "Well, I was cutting an onion and then my eyes began watering so bad I could not see."

Doug, looking very serious, replied: "Well, yes I understand. And how do your eyes feel now?"

The patient replied: "Well, I flushed them out. They kept burning but they feel better now...still stinging a bit.

While this was going on I was doing everything to not laugh. I was actually pretending to cough as I was having difficulty not bursting out laughing. With Doug's serious concerned demeanor and the patient's description it was becoming too much to take to maintain a straight face. I had begun to record the patient's name and details on our form.

Doug continued to conduct his assessment, taking the man's vital signs, looking into his eyes for redness, and checking his vision.

At one point, Doug said: "Are you on any medications?"

The patient replied: "No."

Doug said: "Should you be on any medications?"

At this point I could not control myself, began to fake cough as I was going to burst out laughing. I presumed Doug asked this question as an indirect one, suggesting that he should be medicated for some mental illness.

I said: "I am just going to step outside to get this cough under control, I will be right back."

Doug looked at me with a completely controlled face and said: "I understand."

I was still amazed that he was able to keep a straight face and remain composed during his assessment. I left the home and headed to the ambulance, by the time I entered the cab I was laughing to tears. It was simply too much to remain composed. I laughed for at least five minutes straight. I re-directed my thoughts as I knew I had to get back inside. When I re-entered the house, they were still in the living room area. Doug was trying to convince the patient to come to the hospital.

There was a pause in the conversation and I said: "Where is the onion?"

The patient said: "Do you want to see it?"

Well, this was an opportunity; this call was already completely ridiculous, so I could not resist. I replied: "Yes, can we?"

The patient got up and headed toward the kitchen. I followed, and Doug was close behind me. As we entered the kitchen the patient said, "It's over there," and pointed to the food processor on the counter with a large amount of onion shredded nearby.

I moved ahead of the patient, put my hand out to stop him from walking, and said: "Sir, I will get you to stay back from the offending onion." Inside I was laughing, but outside I was now calm and collected. The patient stopped and looked at me, somewhat confused. Doug, who was just behind him, was grinning from ear to ear at this point. The younger boy was also in the kitchen observing what was happening.

I walked over to the food processor with the shredded onion. I turned to the patient and said: "Sir, do you have any onions in their natural state?"

The patient said, "Yes over in that bowl," pointing to a bowl on the counter.

I moved toward the counter and noticed two yellow onions and one red onion. I said: "So which type of onion were you processing?"

The patient replied: "The yellow onion."

I said with a very serious look: "Well, from now on I would avoid cutting, chopping or otherwise processing yellow onions to avoid this from happening again."

The patient replied "Uh, ok," with a rather confused look on his face.

The younger boy suddenly had a rather dismissive look on his face, turned, and left the kitchen. Doug, who had been quiet until now said: "Yes, we seem to have narrowed it down to the yellow onions, let's go the hospital and get you checked out."

The patient must have suddenly become aware that we were mocking him and perhaps felt rather embarrassed by the entire situation, as he said: "I think I will be ok, so I am just going to stay home."

I said: "We think in our medical opinion that you should come in to get checked out."

The patient again said: "Uh, no, I am staying home."

Doug said: "Well, we will have to get you to sign our release of liability and refusal before we can go."

The patient said: "Sure, whatever."

Doug produced the section of the form and after he signed we departed the residence. We said nothing until we were driving away from the call. I was trying not to laugh again as I thought of the call and situation.

Doug said: "That was too bad. I wanted to take him to the hospital... they would not believe us."

I was laughing again so hard I was having difficulty breathing and replied: "Yeah, you can't make this stuff up!" I continued laughing again, tears coming to my eyes. I even had to pull over at one point as I was unable to see clearly.

Doug looked over at me with a big smile and said: "Do you want me to drive back?"

In between breaths I said: "No, I will be ok...just give me a minute."

The rest of the drive back to the station was uneventful.

The Screamer

My partner and I were sitting at the station when the hotline rang. We were the up car so we headed out to the bay. It was my drive day, but we both looked briefly at the CAD. The call was a for psych patient, Code 3 but we were instructed to wait for the 5s. The bay door was opening, and I fired the car up.

Dispatch called on the radio: "75A3, the call is Code 3 but a wait for the 5s."

I grabbed the mic and said: "75A3 — 10-4."

I headed in the direction of the call, Code 3 only due to the distance. We were approximately twelve minutes away and often the police take a while depending on their proximity to the call. There was no reason to go Code 3 to end up waiting a few blocks away but, due to distance, if the information was not accurate on the CAD and we were needed, we wanted to be as close as possible. Traffic was not too heavy en route and we arrived in the area in less than seven minutes. I turned off the emergency equipment as we turned off a main road approximately two minutes from the call. We noticed a fire pumper sitting in a nearby parking lot of a mall that was a few blocks from the call. We were not sure if they were staged also, or not.

We entered the townhome complex as the CAD had indicated the police were on scene. As we pulled in, the CAD blipped an alert. Just then the dispatcher came on the air: "75A3, police on scene requesting to wait until safe. Possible violent patient."

We were only a short distance from the scene at this point and a man, seeing us, began waving us in frantically. I began to follow him in slowly, even though we were given this new information. I stopped the car and he began shouting at us to come forward.

I leaned out of the window and shouted: "Sir, we have been told to wait back for the police." He looked puzzled and dropped his arms and walked away.

I turned to my partner and said: "I am just going to pull up a bit more, see if we can see the police. They probably forgot we were staged."

My partner Todd said: "Yeah, true enough. We can sit for a while before they clear us to move in."

I pulled the car around the corner of the townhouse complex. We could see the two police cars parked down the laneway. I backed down and stopped about forty feet from the police cars. We both exited the car and walked toward the police cars. There were two officers standing nearby. One of them had a Caucasian female patient cuffed to the rear of her body. The woman, who was probably twenty-seven-years-old, was standing calmly with the two male officers. As we approached, one of the officers said: "We are just waiting for a female member to search her."

Todd said: "OK."

A few moments later, the woman suddenly and without warning screamed out loudly for about thirty seconds.

I stood there a bit puzzled as there was no other person around and her outburst was rather spontaneous and random.

We talked with the officers a bit when a man loomed from the far end of the laneway. The lighting was dim, so we did not see much more than a figure silhouette until he came closer.

As he got within the proximity of the police cars one of the officers said: "Sir, we are going to ask you to stay back. We are dealing with a situation." The man, who was a Caucasian man in his late fifties, said: "I just wanted to see what was going on and if anyone required any assistance."

The police officer replied: "We have it under control."

The man, still walking toward the scene and now thirty feet away said: "I live here and wanted to hear what all the commotion was about."

At that moment, my normally calm partner got rather agitated, moved toward the man a bit (twenty feet away), and said in a loud voice: "The situation is under control. Can't you see that? The police are here and managing the situation. You have been told to stay back. What do you think you are going to do to help out? The police are handling it!!" He was very agitated.

I chuckled a bit; hearing him get so annoyed at this man was very funny to me at this point.

I said to Todd: "I am going to wait in the car until the other member arrives."

He replied, "Sure, OK," still sounding annoyed.

I walked back to the car and climbed in, as it was chilly out. Todd came back into the car and looked over at me and said: "Can you believe that guy? Walking up wanting to help... what the fuck is wrong with him anyway?"

I was laughing now, as I listened to him express his discontent.

Todd looked over at me, almost glaring now and said: "Well...don't you agree?"

I replied, "I do agree...just funny...you are always so chill, then you just explode on this guy," laughing again and smiling.

The woman had a few more random spontaneous screaming events before the female officer finally showed up and searched the woman for any sharp objects or weapons. Due to the woman's erratic state, we decided to follow the police to the hospital rather than place the woman in the back of our Ambulance. We did what we call a medical escort. If there is an issue the police will pull over and we will intervene and deal with any medical issues. The call ended without incident.

The Doctor who did not do home repair

We were enjoying some much-needed downtime at the station. It was early in the morning (0430) and we had been working steadily most of the evening. The hotline rang — I am not sure how they managed to make that ring the most annoying ring sound ever. These phones are the old-style phones that cradle in a moveable base; there is no dial pad simply a large, bulky handset. The phones are red, of course, identifying them as a hotline.

My partner answered the phone. It was a stabbing with both ALS and ourselves. I had a student this block so when he heard of the call he was jacked up. This type of call is very exciting for the students, as we all want exciting calls in this line of work. These are the calls that get our blood moving and motivate us to do our job and motivate us for the less exciting calls we do, as those calls are the bulk of our work.

We departed the station together with the ALS, driving off-set down the road to clear traffic. There were few cars on the road as it was early. The emergency lights flashed against the roadway and signs as we sped to the call. The call was a wait for the police when we left the station – we would wait a few blocks away and "stage" until it was safe to enter, in case there were other violent threats still present. On the way to the call the CAD message changed and indicated it was "safe – police on scene."

When we arrived, there were a few police cars and the Fire Department was already on scene. We grabbed our kit and O2 and headed up to the call. It was a run-down house; the twenty or more stairs up the house were in a poor state of repair and looked like they would break on every step.

I entered the home first with my student; the ALS paramedic followed behind with the remaining crew members. There were three firefighters in the room and two police officers. The man who was stabbed was sitting on the couch, his entire t-shirt covered in blood.

I noticed a tourniquet on his right arm as I moved in toward his left side. I could see stab wounds to both arms. I grabbed my super scissors from my duty belt and began cutting his shirt off to expose his chest, abdomen and back. The other ALS Paramedic was also examining the patient. He was talking and conscious, telling us it hurt. (In my mind I thought, 'You think?' He was stabbed multiple times; I guess it hurt). After exposing his chest, back and abdomen we found no life-threatening stab wounds; most were to his arms, legs and non-vital areas. He was extricated to our cot down the stairs and loaded into the ALS Ambulance. There was some discussion and I ended up driving them to the nearby trauma centre less than fifteen minutes away. I drove Code 3 but very smoothly, watching the crew in the back from the rear cabin camera, where I could see everything that they were doing, including standing up during the transport. The ALS Paramedic notified the hospital via cell what we were coming in with.

When we arrived at the trauma centre, we were directed to Trauma Bay #1. The patient was moved to his bed and the team of nurses and other techs began to cut his clothing off, apply monitors, draw blood and begin recording information.

I left the trauma bay after the ALS paramedic gave report to the staff and ER doctor. I then began to clean the Ambulance and cot, and replace equipment used on the call. It was determined that he had eight non-life-threatening stab wounds to his body. My student stayed in the trauma bay to watch for a bit while the staff removed our dressings and began charting the wounds.

After the Ambulance was cleaned, mopped, and ready for another call, I walked back to the trauma bay with my student to see how things were going with the patient. When we entered, the ER physician was gowned with a facemask and shield on, was wearing surgical gloves and had a suture tray to his right. He looked over as he entered.

The doctor said: "Hi."

I replied: "Hi, I saw you at Starbucks on my way to work. I would have said 'hi' but you looked busy."

The doctor said: "Yeah I saw you also. I was in town as my son has violin lessons and we had to make a Cabela's visit while in town."

I replied: "Yes, I understand that. So how do his wounds look?"

The doctor replied: "Well, his bicep muscle is intact." (As he said this, he was digging into the 6cm-long gaping wound to the patient's right arm with his finger).

I then began to absorb the scene: the man was laying on the trauma bed table; he was conscious, and his wounds were all exposed; his left arm with two wounds approximately 2-3cm were dripping blood and it was pooling in a small pool on the floor; the other wounds were not seeping blood as much but were still exposed.

The doctor then picked up a suture staple gun and began stapling the man's wound shut from the bottom up. I heard "Clink, clink," as he held the skin together and placed another stable. Each time the doctor placed a staple, the patient would say: "Ow!"

The Doctor continued and on his fourth staple he stopped and said: "Ah, that is why I don't do home repair!" He looked over to his suture tray and said: "Now where are my forceps?"

One of the RNs in the room said: "I have one here if you need it."

He found one in the tray and replied: "That's OK, I have one here." He grabbed the staple that didn't connect the two sides of the tissue and pulled it out with a quick tug. As he did so the patient again exclaimed: "Ow!"

I said: "I have never seen a staple put in a wound on the arm before."

The doctor replied: "Yeah, I should have been done by now."

The doctor picked up the staple gun again and began stapling again. Each time he placed a staple the man would say "Ow," and each time the patient said "Ow" the doctor would chuckle: "He he."

After a couple more staples, the doctor again stopped, said "Ahh," picked up the forceps, and removed the poorly-placed staple; again, the man said "Ow" followed by the doctor chuckling: "He he."

It took everything for me not to break out laughing in the trauma room. Here was a guy who had been stabbed eight times, lying in the trauma room, leaking blood on the floor, as the ER doctor sutures his arm with a staple gun and is missing a few of the staples as he is going, chuckling each time the patient says 'Ow.' This was literally hilarious to me.

We left the trauma room and headed back to the Ambulance to meet up with my partner and head back to our station for crew change.

Time for coffee

My regular partner (Todd) and I had been assigned a call for a man who was walking around the neighbourhood with bloody hands. It was a wait for the police. We had staged a few blocks away out of sight and after waiting ten minutes we decided to get a much-needed coffee at the Tim Hortons – I don't like the coffee at Tim Hortons and normally would drink a Starbucks, but they began offering shots of espresso for 70 cents, so I started to stop in on occasion for a couple shots. The Tims was only a block from us. My partner parked in the parking lot and we walked in with our portables on in case we were given the 'safe to move in' instructions.

It was not very busy but seemed to take forever for the staff to process the three people at the counter. As we stood next in line, I felt a poke in my back. I turned and a man in a transit bus driver uniform was standing there.

He said: "Hey, there is a guy in the bushes out there not moving."

I replied: "Oh?" with a look of little concern on my face.

He said: "You should go check him out."

I replied: "Maybe he is just sleeping."

He replied: "Well, he is not moving."

I replied: "That's what happens when we sleep. Someone will call it in. Did you call 911?"

He said: "No I didn't. I actually just wanted to get ahead of you two in line as I am in a rush...ha ha."

I replied: "Well, we didn't start this job yesterday. Besides, we are actually on a standby call with the police right now" I laughed.

My partner who had been listening said, "Yeah, we have been doing this for a while now...takes more than that to get us to respond," laughing now as well.

The bus driver said: "Well, I feel like I am going to fall asleep if I don't get a coffee to give me a pick me up. This line is sure moving slow."

I replied: "What time are you off?"

He replied: "Twelve."

I glanced down at my watch and noticed it was just before 2200hrs.

After a few more minutes that seemed like hours to be next in line, the bus driver said: "I am going to have to go soon if they don't hurry up."

Moments later, the line moved ahead, and the bus driver looked at me with a glance of anticipation.

I said: "Go ahead."

He replied: "Really? Thanks, that's great!"

I said, "No problem," as I looked over at my partner, who nodded and smiled.

We eventually got our two-shot expressos and, as we were leaving, our radios crackled: "75A3, you are safe to move in. Police on scene."

I grabbed my mike and said: "10-4."

As we walked back to the car, Todd said, "That bus driver sure didn't know what to do when we didn't jump to it, when he told us about the man down," chuckling.

I replied: "Yeah, I know. It was pretty funny neither one of us even flinched. You know you have been working this area too long when..."

Todd said: "Yeah, no kidding."

We got into our car and headed over to the call we were assigned to. Apparently, a man walking around with blood-covered hands. The neighbours thought that was suspicious so called the police. Yes, that is not odd at all — walking around the neighbourhood with hands covered in blood!

We attended the call and the man had broken his glass living room table; there was some sort of mental illness involved. We cleaned up his wounds and left him in the care of the police. Just another day on the job.

Time for a break

We had been at the station and were second car down so Todd and I decided to go across the street to the Tim Hortons for a coffee. Knowing that we would get a call if we just went on available vehicle, Todd called the dispatcher as we drove over to give him heads up we were technically down car, so A2 should get the call before us.

After Todd hung up I said: "You know though that if we get an echo or serious delta call we will be getting it."

Todd replied: "Yeah, oh well. Let's just see what happens. This is a good dispatcher tonight."

I said: "Yes, sounds good...I need some caffeine."

I was driving tonight, I would normally have a Starbucks but now that Tim's was serving the espresso shots, it was possible to have a good coffee there. After we parked and began walking toward the door, we heard ambulance sirens coming from the station. An ambulance entered the intersection just as I walked into the Tims, so I never noticed the direction it was going.

Todd said: "Well, there goes Alpha 2."

We walked in and there was a line of about five people; not bad, but a delay nonetheless. After ordering, Todd said: "Hey, who is that?"

I looked outside the window that viewed the street and could see flashing red and white lights. It was an ambulance on a call right at Tim Hortons. In my mind I thought: 'Why would a car be dispatched to where we were getting a coffee? Why did the dispatcher not call us on the portable?'

I had just paid and said to Todd: "I am going to head outside see if they need a hand." I thought it must not be too serious a call if we had not been contacted.

Todd replied: "OK, I will be right out also."

I excited the Tims and, as I walked over, noticed it was our Alpha 2 car. There was a power wheelchair and they were feverishly working on assessing a patient. A bit surprised, I said: "Hey Calvin, do you need some help?"

Calvin looked up, a bit surprised: "Oh hey Luch. Yeah, can you draw up some Narcan?" He was working on the airway and his partner was handing him the BVM. "Where did you come from?" he asked me.

I replied: "We were inside ordering coffee. I can't believe the dispatcher didn't call us on our radio."

Calvin said: "Yeah, no kidding. So this woman ODed. Just going to get her sats up before we give the Narcan. She was sating at 47% SPO2 when we arrived. We pulled her out of her chair and just started working on her when you walked out."

I opened their kit and grabbed a multi-dose of Narcan as well as a 3cc 22g 1/1/2" needle. I said: "Calvin, do you want 0.8?"

Calvin said: "Sure 0.8. She seems pretty down. Just going to wait a few minutes to get her sats up to 100%. They are 95% now."

I looked over at the SPO2 monitor and it read '95' in bright red LED numbers on the screen; I also noticed her pulse was racing at 135bpm.

Calvin's partner appeared to be new, just based on how excited he was; he appeared a bit unsure of himself in his actions and mannerisms. Just then, the fire department arrived — a three-man crew including a captain. I recognized this crew as we had worked on many calls together.

I said: "Calvin, do you want me to give the Narcan now?"

Calvin replied: "No, hold off Luch. I want to get her sats up for a bit before we give it."

I said: "Sure, just let me know."

I chatted with the FD for a bit then noticed my partner Todd walk out of Tim Hortons with a coffee and some food. He joined the conversation.

Calvin said: "OK Luch — you can give the Narcan now."

I said "OK," exposed the woman's upper arm, injected the needle, and administered the 0.8mg Narcan."

A few minutes later, a woman from the Tim Hortons came outside holding a coffee. She looked over at me and smiled. She said: "This is your coffee."

I replied: "OK, sure. Can you just place it on the window ledge?" She smiled and placed the coffee on the outer window ledge. At this point I realized how odd it was that we were in the middle of dealing with an OD and my coffee I had purchased was being brought out to me. It was very nice of the staff to do that of course; it just seemed so odd as it has never happened to me before.

Calvin was stimulating the woman with a sternal rub to wake her up, as it had been over two minutes since the injection. Normally, if the person only took heroin (as opposed to Fentanyl), 0.4-0.8 IM works enough to get them conscious. She began to groan and opened her eyes; she tried to sit up immediately which is very common when people OD for some reason. The BVM and OPA was removed as she woke up.

We spoke to the woman about her OD, and she admitted to having ODed a couple of times in the past. We assisted her into her wheelchair, but she declined coming to the hospital for monitoring as most of our OD victims do. We cleaned up the scene of all our equipment and headed back to our car. As soon as we cleared, another call was dropped on our CAD.

The Glock

It was a regular, steady day on car, with no exciting calls yet. To a paramedic the exciting calls are ones that are usually very traumatic for the persons involved. We simply want to challenge our skills to the limit; we perhaps even want to save a life on occasion. That is what drives us: the unknown; the adrenaline rush of blasting into harm's way to make a difference; the thrill of making snap judgement decisions when time is often critical and seconds count.

We had just cleared a call and were nearby a Home Depot. I told my partner I wanted to stop in to use the washroom. It was my drive day, so I parked as close as possible near the entrance, placed us on portable, and made my way inside. The washrooms were of course at the back of the store. As soon as I walked in, I heard the dispatcher call us.

Dispatch: "75A3."

I grabbed my mike and replied: "75A3."

Dispatch: "75A3 on portable, 75A3."

I depressed my mike button again and replied: "75A3." The radio made a beep sound indicating that the transmission didn't get out.

I quickly relieved myself of my full bladder and headed out of the washroom. I felt my phone vibrate. I looked at it and read the text from my partner waiting outside: "We have a call." I knew this of course and quickly walked out of the store.

I got to the car and quickly jumped into the driver's seat.

My partner said: "We have a shooting!"

I replied: "Oh, where is it?"

My partner said: "Just head out and turn left and up Dawns road. It's about ten minutes from here."

I replied, "Maybe eight the way I drive," smiling now.

I flipped all the emergency lights on, and as I exited the driveway from the Home Depot I turned on the siren. Once on the main road,

I pressed the accelerator to the floor and the engine roared at the strain as I began to accelerate. I said: "Do we have ALS?"

My partner replied: "Yes, they are a bit closer. They might beat us there."

I said: "Not if I can help it."

I pushed it as I drove to this call, driving faster than I normally do, using precision driving to navigate into oncoming traffic to bypass the common medians near intersections. We were only three minutes from the call when the radio squawked:

25A1: "It's a confirmed Code 4."

Dispatch: "10-4 confirmed Code 4."

Dispatch: "75A3, you can cancel. Cancelled by crew on scene."

I said: "Like hell we are cancelled — this is the most interesting call we have done all week. We are going." I continued driving Code 3 toward the call, now only a few minutes away.

Dispatch: "75A3 did you copy the cancel?"

My partner said: "Funny how we can't hear the radio sometimes."

I replied: "Yes, sometimes I accidentally hit the volume and it lowers the volume. With the siren you can't actually hear the radio anymore, weird." My partner smiled.

S10 (in an aggressive tone): "This is S10. 75A3, you are cancelled!'"

. I thought in my head, 'Oh, he is pissed we are not answering our radio and trying to intimidate us with his supervisor role. Well I have been around a while and he can't prove we didn't answer the radio.'

As we pulled up a few moments later, we saw three police cars and the ALS unit. I pulled behind the ALS unit, grabbed my reflective vest, and carefully exited the car. I could smell the burnt-like smell from the brakes from all the heavy braking on the way to the call as I walked toward a police officer. There was a small group of Indo-Canadians nearby all crying and upset.

She said: "The other crew is over there."

I nodded and noticed a narrow trail that lead into the bushes. I walked up the short, steep incline of dirt, brushing past the brush that lined the narrow trail. I walked a short twenty-five feet and arrived to find a few police officers and the ALS crew. One of the members was connecting ECG leads to the victim. He was laying on his back, but I could not see his face at this time.

The ALS paramedic saw me and said: "Hey Luch."

I replied: "Hey Don."

I noticed the black steel of a Glock semi-automatic handgun laying nearby. I moved in a bit closer to the victim and, upon seeing his face and head, was surprised to see the bottom of his jaw was missing, as well as a portion of his face; it was a grizzly image. It appeared he had committed suicide by placing the handgun under his mouth.

I said: "So, suicide?"

A female police officer standing nearby replied: "Yes, and his family that is out on the roadway found him. He had been missing for two days."

I said: "Oh, wow, that is why they were so upset."

I walked back to the roadway; the family was in tears, hugging each other. As I walked to the Ambulance I thought to myself, 'How was it possible that his car was parked on a busy road for two days and no police checked it? I suppose that unless it was reported missing, or an officer passed by the vehicle over the course of those two days, why would they check the car?' It just seemed odd that the victim was less than fifty feet from the road and lied there dead with a loaded handgun at his side.

I got back inside the car. My partner came back a few moments later, entered the cab, and sat down. I was chilly out and, since there was nothing for us to do, we would be clearing shortly. Just then, a supervisor arrived at my partner's window; she was not the one who had made the radio broadcast earlier to cancel.

She said: "Did you see the body?"

My partner replied: "Yes."

She looked over at us with concern on her face and said: "Are you OK?'

I looked at her and said: "Yes, I am, thanks for asking. We are going to clear shortly."

She looked at my partner and said: "Are you OK? If you guys need any CIS let me know."

My partner replied: "No, I'm good."

She almost didn't seem to believe us and said: "Well, if you need any support let me know."

I replied: "Sure, thanks for that."

After she walked away my partner said: "Well, she certainly was being concerned about how we are."

I replied: "Yeah, well, guess it's good; better than offering no support like they used to years ago. In the past they would just be asking us to clear to head to another call."

My partner replied: "No kidding."

I said: "Let's take a few more minutes, then clear. I have to make a quick call."

My partner replied: "Sure, sounds good."

Emergency landing

I was working de-paired on an ALS car. It was a dayshift and had worked on this car in the past. We were having a steady day but nothing shattering so far. Suddenly the CAD sounded: "Blip...blip...blip."

My partner, Adrian, looked at the CAD and said: "Oh, we have an aircraft emergency at Button Airport." I spun the CAD to take a quick look and it read:

- Location: Airport
- Response: Code 3
- Type: Aircraft Emergency
- Call source: ATC
- Units: 39A1, 83A2, S10
- Remarks: Pilot unable to lower landing gear. Cessna 210, 1 person on board, unable to lower gear. 40min ETA to Button airport.

I replied: "This could be interesting." I activated the emergency lights and siren and began our response to the airport. It was a clear day and sunny — a beautiful day to fly, I thought. We arrived at the airport just as the other BLS unit, 83A2, arrived. They were sitting at the gate near the tower. I pulled up and we talked a bit about access to the airport. The local city FD was supposed to arrive but there was some confusion about what runway the aircraft was going to be landing on and where we should stage. We did not have the ATC frequency on our radios, so we could not talk to them. We also did not have their phone number.

I keyed the mike and said: "39A1."

Dispatch: "39A1."

I said: "39A1, we are at the main gate by the tower. It is locked. We do not have access to airside. Are there any airport personnel going to give us access to the apron?"

Dispatch: "Standby 39A1. Will get back to you."

Adrian said: "Well, we are not going to be very good on this side of the fence."

I replied: "Well, we can probably access the apron on the other side. I was here a week ago and the gate was closed but not locked. We could check it out and see if we can gain access while Dispatch gets back to us."

Adrian said: "Sure, let's check it out."

I drove down to the next access road, past a number of hangars, and down a road toward the gate. I got out and checked the gate: it was unlocked. I opened the gate and got back into the Ambulance. Adrian said: "Great. We should let Dispatch know we have gained access to airside."

I drove through the gate, stopped, got out, and closed the gate behind me. I then grabbed the mike and said: "39A1."

Dispatch: "39A1."

I said: "39A1 we were able to access airside via a small gate on the south side. Were you able to get in touch with the tower to find out the staging point and runway being used?"

Dispatch: "We were not able to get in direct contact with the tower, but you are advised to stage at the end of Runway 25."

I thought about this for a minute, then said to Adrian: "Runway 25...that is on the far end of the airport. We will have to drive all the way around to the other road and then be behind a locked gate again."

Adrian replied: "Yeah, does not make a lot of sense. Let's just stage here for a bit until we get better confirmation."

I said: "Yeah, OK. I'm going to see if I can contact the tower directly. If I can't find the number, I have the direct number to the tower in Abbotsford, so perhaps they can transfer me or give me the number direct to the tower."

Adrian replied: "Sure, go for it; we seem to be in the dark at the moment."

After trying to find the direct number to the tower at Button airport with no luck, I called the tower at Abbotsford Airport. I spoke to the controller and explained we were an ambulance on standby for an aircraft emergency. He was able to give me the number for the tower at Button airport. I then called them and they were relieved as the local city fire department had not yet been in touch with them on the designated air frequency so they had no contact with us on the apron. I was told to stage just past the tower on the apron, clear of the active runway. I was given updated information on the location of the aircraft and what he planned to do including which runway based on the current surface winds. While I spoke to him our S10 supervisor had showed up. We gave him access to the apron as well as the other BLS unit that had gone to the other side of the airport after we had spoken initially. We all staged at the staging point. The local city Fire Department was also on scene. On the radio I heard that an MSU was also on the way, as was a CCT ambulance. We were standing outside of our ambulances on the apron, and I was giving verbal update to S10 as I was the only one with direct contact with the tower.

I was standing next to the S10 (Harry) and said: "Isn't there a lot of resources arriving for a single pilot in a small aircraft?"

Harry replied: "Yes, I would agree. Think everyone just wants to be part of the action and they are not on calls."

I said: "OK, well, just seems that an ALS, BLS and yourself is plenty; having an MSU and CCT...bit overkill." I laughed.

Harry replied: "Yup, I agree."

Within a short time, the other ambulances that had indicated they would respond were on scene and positioned themselves in a row below the tower. The tower called me every five minutes or so to give me an update, and the tower operator asked me why there were so many ambulances on scene. I simply told them they were available and perhaps wanted to see what was happening, as I did not have a logical reply for her.

In a short time, the Cessna 210 came in to do a low overflight over the runway. He had plenty of fuel, so he wanted to make sure of his approach prior to landing. I assumed the whole time, being a pilot with twenty-four years of experience, that he would do a no-gear landing on the grass beside the runway, as there was no chance of sparks and it was softer than the hard surface.

After the pilot did two low overflights of the runway we were told that he would, in fact, land on a different runway, one that was in close proximity to where we were staged and provided better access if there was a crash.

Harry turned to Adrian and myself and said: "So you guys are going to be the only car going out on the runway after the Fire Department deem it safe...well, and myself." He said this with a grin. Harry wanted to be part of the action as well and, as a supervisor, had some privileges.

Adrian turned to me and said: "Hey, there was a reason we were de-paired today. Your pilot background certainly made this more seamless by contacting the tower. Dispatch was not giving us very much info."

The tower finally notified me via the cell phone that the Cessna was going to attempt a landing. He came in perfectly with the partially retracted rear landing gear, but to my horror he was settling over the hard surface runway that was paved. My main thought was: 'When he lands there could be sparks from the metal scraping across the runway. With high-octane aviation fuel the chance of a fire and or explosion is possible.'

The aircraft slowly descended onto the surface of the runway. The front landing gear looked fully down. As the aircraft touched down, we could hear the scraping of the gear as the aircraft caused it to collapse, and the fuselage scraped on the runway surface. There were a few sparks initially, then the plane came to a stop, resting on the left-wing tip. The front landing gear remained down. The Fire Department immediately headed toward the aircraft, emergency lights on. I pulled in behind them, maintaining distance in case there was a fire or explosion. When the Fire Department had a charged hose, we moved in. The pilot, who was the sole occupant of the plane, was standing beside the plane, assessing the damage. I pulled up at a safe distance and walked over to the pilot with my partner. The pilot was not injured and was on a bit of an emotional high from a very safe, stable landing.

After we took a few photos, we departed the runway and made our way back toward the apron where the remaining emergency vehicles were stationed. As I drove back, I noticed three police cars, two fire trucks and three ambulances, plus a paramedic supervisor vehicle. I thought again that this was a lot of resources for a small plane with only the pilot on board.

As we drove back Adrian said: "Well, he did a pretty good landing, all considered."

I replied: "Yes very impressive. I am still amazed he landed on the hard surface versus the grass to the side."

Adrian said: "Well, maybe he was concerned the front gear would dig in and cause the plane to flip."

I replied: "Yes, perhaps. I know I would have opted for the softer grass and no hazard risk of sparks if it was me. Guess a judgement call that he made. Perfect landing from my view though; very skilled pilot."

Adrian said: "Yes, agreed."

Diabetic NPA

We had just cleared a call and the CAD sounded: "Blip...blip...blip!" I spun the CAD and it read:

- Location: 3456 Sutton Rd Anytown
- Response: Code 3
- Type: Unconscious/Diabetic history
- Call source: Person on scene
- Units: 77A1
- Remarks: Patient is an insulin dependent diabetic

I spun it back to my partner to see the address. I said: "Looks like a possible hypoglycaemic."

My partner, "Joe," replied: "It sure does."

I was attending today and my partner Joe was driving. It was early morning, approximately 1:00a.m. We are dispatched to an unconscious man with a diabetic history. My partner lit it up and we started to head toward the call located at a residence. We arrived to find the local fire department on scene. I said: "I hope they have not pushed a bunch of glucogel into his mouth. They always do that before we arrive, and it just causes airway issues and does not absorb enough to actually raise the patient's blood glucose. Wish they would hold off a few minutes until we arrive so we can treat them quickly and effectively...sigh."

When we entered the residence, we were met by a family member who led us into a bedroom. As I walked through the door, I could see a queen-sized bed in a room that was a bit too small for it to fit properly; there were two Fire members over the side of the bed. I went around to see them squeezing glucogel into the unconscious man's mouth as he was on his side, wedged against the wall and the bed, lying on the floor.

I said: "Hey, guys. Stop with the glucogel, OK?"

The fireman who had been squeezing the glucogel tube into his mouth looked back at me and replied: "Uh, ok."

I said: "Let's move him onto the bed."

The two firefighters, myself, and my partner moved this rather large man onto the bed. As we struggled with his dead weight, I thought: 'Why do they always have to be big guys that have to be lifted and moved?'

After we had him on his back on the bed and I had moved into access his LOC, I said: "What is his name?"

The family member replied: "His name is Fred."

As I pinched his trapezius at his shoulder, I said loudly: "Fred... Fred...I'm a Paramedic we are here to help you." There was no response to my efforts to rouse him. I could see he was breathing, and moved to check his carotid pulse — it was present — then I moved to check his radial pulse; it was weak and fast.

My partner, Joe, had already opened the kit, and was accessing the equipment we would need to manage the unconscious man. I looked over at Joe and said: "Hey can you hand me a red airway?"

Joe replied, "Sure," as he handed me a red OPA.

I said: "How did he get to the floor? Was it a fall?"

The family member replied: "I came in and found him on the floor, so I don't know." I thought about his for a moment and considered that a person who is asleep rolling off a bed is low risk for a neck injury.

I positioned Fred's head backwards and looked into his airway; there was gooey, sticky glucogel in his mouth and around his lips.

I said: "Joe, can you hand me the suction? I have to suction a bit of this glucogel before I insert the airway." Joe handed me the yanker suction handle and I inserted it into the man's mouth. It was a challenge, as the man's jaw was seized so would not open all the way. The 'hummmm' of the suction could be heard, as well as the sucking sound as I moved the tip around his mouth to remove the glucogel. I thought to myself: 'Sometimes I hate first responders. They knew we were arriving and they had to start putting this crap in his mouth even though they know we start IVs to treat diabetics. Uhg. I know they mean well, but we arrived a few minutes after them, I am sure they heard our siren.'

After I was done suctioning, I sized and tried to insert the OPA; it would not go in. I tried to open his jaw, but no luck — he had trismus.

I looked at Joe and said: "Hey, can you hand me the pack of NPAs? This guy is not accepting an OPA. His jaw has trismus."

Joe replied, "You bet," and handed me a pack of five NPAs so that I could find the right size. I looked and grabbed one of the biggest ones, sized it, lubed it with the small lubricant package, and taped to the side of the airway.

One of the firemen said: "Wow that is a big airway!"

I began to insert it into the patient's left nostril, twisting it slightly from side to side as I did. It went in easily, leaving the rubber flange with the opening at the nose.

I replied: "Yeah it is, but this is a big guy, and the right size. I have never used the largest size yet actually."

A soon as I was done, my partner, who was already thinking ahead, handed me a O2 mask; the pulse oximeter was already on Fred's finger and it read 89%. I placed the mask over his face.

Joe had already opened the blood glucose test kit and was getting ready to take a sample from his finger. I scanned Fred's body: He was wearing a t-shirt and sweat pants and he was incontinent of urine; the unpleasant acrid odour filled the room. There were no obvious injuries on his body.

I looked down at the pulse oximeter and it now read 98%. Joe had just obtained a blood sample and the glucose meter sounded off with a 'beep' indicating that the test was done.

Joe said: "Sugar is 1.2."

I replied: "That explains why he is so down. Can you prime a line of D10 and I will look for access?"

Joe said: "Already on it."

I always liked when I worked with seasoned partners who were already a step ahead of the call; often little talking was required as we knew what had to be done.

I grabbed an IV start kit, applied a blue rubber tourniquet to his upper arm at the bicep and began looking for a vein. A couple began to pop out, one at his AC and another on his forearm. I wanted to put in at least an 18g catheter in case he also needed fluids or there were other complications beyond low blood glucose. I swabbed the arm with an alcohol swab, prepared my 18g IV catheter, anchored his skin and inserted it. The blood filled the entry chamber, confirming entry into the vein. I advanced the catheter to the hub, retracted the needle, and popped the tourniquet off with the other hand. I placed a piece of tegaderm over the catheter; when I looked up Joe had the IV tubing ready and handed it to me. I connected it and said: "OK, you can open it up." Joe opened the IV flow adjustment to full drip rate, then motioned a firefighter to hold the IV bag for him.

I looked at the Fire Captain and said: "Cap, would you mind getting our cot out and setting it up for egress? I want to get this guy going as soon as possible."

The Fire Captain replied: "Sure, I will get my guys on it."

I said: "Great, thanks."

Joe said: "Do you still want ALS?"

I replied: "Yes, until this guy wakes up, better keep them coming."

Joe said: "Agreed."

After 300ml of D10W flowed into the man, with still no response from him, I leaned closer to him, squeezed his trapezius and shouted: "Fred, can you hear me? I am a paramedic here to help you." There was no response.

I grabbed the glucose meter and took another sample of blood; I read the screen and it showed a reading of 2.4. I looked at Joe and said: "This guy is only at 2.4 and we have given 300ml already. Most people would be up, talking to us by now. He must have been down for a while." The family had told us that he had gone to bed a few hours earlier and it was not until they heard the 'thud' of him rolling off the bed that they checked on him and found him unresponsive. It appeared to be over five hours, so if his blood glucose was that low he could have sustained some brain injury.

Just as the IV bag was almost empty, with still not response, an ALS crew walked in. I knew the attending paramedic and gave him the report. I said: "Hey Stewart, this man was found down, beside his bed unresponsive, last seen about five hours ago. He is an insulin-dependent diabetic and his initial sugar was 1.2. We administered 300ml of D10W with no cognitive response and took another sugar; it was 2.4. As you can see, we have emptied the 500ml bag and still have no response. I was just about to take another sugar."

Stewart said: "OK. See you have the cot ready. Let's check his sugar. I am going to draw up some D50. Let's get him on the cot in the meantime and I will administer it before we leave. Are we suspecting a CVA?"

I replied: "Well there is no CVA or TIA history, but it is possible. I wanted to get his sugars back to normal before started to look for other possible causes."

Stewart said: "Yes, agree. Let's get him on the cot. Maybe we can fore-and-aft him?"

I replied: "Sure, we have enough people." I looked around the room at the firefighters and they all nodded in approval.

I quickly took a blood glucose and it read 3.0. I was again surprised that, after all the D10W we gave, his body was simply using it up as fast as we were administering it.

With four of us, we lifted the man and carried him to the doorway where the cot was positioned. Stewart, who had the D50, connected it to the IV and administered it.

We loaded him into the back of the Ambulance and headed off to the local hospital that was only eight minutes away. On the way, Fred called the hospital and spoke to the triage nurse, giving them heads up we would need a resuscitation bed. By the time we were backing up, Fred began waking up. He was very confused, but was able to open his eyes; however, he was unable to say anything at this point. We offloaded him, and he was placed in a trauma bed where a team of three nurses came in to begin assessment and connect him to the monitors, as Stewart gave a verbal report.

After we transferred him to the trauma bed and moved our cot and equipment out of the room, we talked a bit about the call. Joe, Stewart and myself had never seen a diabetic so low that it took 500cc of D10W and D50 to get a response. After the cot was cleaned up, I went back to the trauma room to see how Fred was doing. I walked in and he was now sitting up in the trauma bed, alert, but looking a bit confused. He was talking rapidly. I almost began laughing though as he still had the huge, green NPA inserted into his left nostril; he did not remove it, nor did the nurses taking care of him. It was just a funny sight to see him talking wide eyed and moving his head all about with this green nasal airway in his nose. I talked with him a few moments, wished him well, and left the trauma room.

Glossary of terms

#9 – A light, portable stretcher, that folds in half. It is made of aluminum tubing covered by a strong rubber type material. It is used to transport patients in fixed wing aircraft or rotary aircraft that are not designated air ambulances.

45A2, 35A1, etc. – Call sign of Ambulance, all letters are pronounced with phonetic alphabet (Alpha, Bravo, Charlie, Delta, Echo etc.)

AC – Antecubital fossa

ACP – Advanced Care Paramedic. PCP is minimum entry into the ACP program and an additional two years of training, plus internship. Trained in advanced medical care assessments, use of cardiac monitor, as well as a wide array of cardiac medications, analgesics, and sedatives.

AED – Automated External Defibrillator. Applied for suspected cardiac arrest patients; will analyze two shockable rhythms and deliver a shock once the shock button is pressed.

AMA – Against Medical Advice

Ambulance – A box van style vehicle, with dual wheels on rear. Used to respond to, treat and transport sick or injured people to the hospital and is capable of carrying a least one stretcher. It is clearly marked and has multiple emergency lights and strobes on various parts of the vehicle. It is equipped with a siren for emergency responses.

Auscultate – Placing a stethoscope over specific areas on the back or chest to listen to breath sounds. This helps determine if the breath sounds are normal or abnormal, aiding in determining the condition and or treatments necessary.

Bay – The covered parking spot where the Ambulance parks, enclosed by a roll-up door.

Bus (jargon) – See 'Ambulance.'

BVM – Bag Valve Mask. Device used to ventilate a patient by placing the mask portion on the patient's face and squeezing a bag to inflate the patient's lungs.

C- Spine – The act of applying a collar and/or clam shell to secure a patient with possible spinal injuries prior to transport.

CAD – Computerized Automated Dispatch. A system that sends a call to a computer-type screen with information on a call including the address and particulars relating to the call.

Call – An assignment given to a crew to respond to an event or incident requiring medical attention by Paramedics.

Canadian Coast Guard Hovercraft Unit – A Canadian Coast Guard unit located on the West coast of British Columbia that uses air cushioned vehicles (hovercraft) to respond to SAR calls or perform other related Coast Guard tasks, as required. The unit has seven rescue specialists, including rescue divers and two officers (one captain, and one first officer who pilot the hovercraft).

Car (jargon) – See 'Ambulance.'

CCP – Critical Care Paramedic – Four-year program. ACP entry requirements are a minimum. They are trained in further advanced drugs, use of pumps, and ventilators, and are normally attached to fixed or rotary aircraft and conduct critical transfers or fly in directly to serious accidents.

Chair cot – A device that looks like a chair with wheels when opened. It has straps that cross the chest and hips, as well as a foot rest with strap. It has a T-bar that extends up as well as a deployable track system that is locked into place to glide the chair cot down stairs with resistance to assist the crew in keeping it from running away. There are extendable hand arms at the bottom and the device is designed as a two-person device. There is an extendable IV pole on the side and deployable folding handles to the rear to assist in steering or lifting, depending on the circumstances. It is stored, folded, at the side door of the ambulance. It is made of tubular aluminum and hard plastic with four swivel wheels at the base.

Clam Shell – Also known as a 'ROS' (Roberson Orthopedic Stretcher). Device that is made in two halves that are clicked together at the head and feet; adjustable in length based on patient size and height and is placed under the patient's entire body. It is a lifting device used to stabilize patients with suspected c-spine injuries, hip fractures, or lower leg fractures. It has six straps that are connected to the device and are criss-crossed at the chest and pelvis area. It is made of tubular aluminum and hard plastic that is designed to slip under the patient with minimal movement.

Code 1 – Unauthorized persons listening to radio transmissions.

Code 2 – Routine response; no lights or sirens; must obey all traffic laws.

Code 3 – Emergency Response; lights and sirens.

Code 4 – Deceased at the scene (not viable for resuscitation efforts)

Code 5 – Police

Code 6 – Fire Department

Code 9 – Infectious patient

Collar – Stiff collar that is adjustable in size from no-neck to tall for adult. There are also child and pediatric collars. They are designed to help splint the neck in the neutral position, protecting the body from movement and further damage.

Cot – Ambulance stretcher

CPAP – Continuous Positive Airway Pressure. A full-face mask that is attached to a patient's face and is designed to help keep the alveoli more filled to allow better oxygenation. Its use has specific criteria based on the paramedic administering it. Its application is to assist persons to breathe and increase oxygenation to the body. Medications such as Ventolin (salbutamol) may also be administered through this device.

CPR – Cardio Pulmonary Resuscitation. Act of compressing on the chest to circulate blood and ventilate the patient to maintain circulating blood flow until advanced resuscitation procedures can be employed.

D10W – 10% dextrose in water. IV solution. Normally given to diabetic patients to treat hypoglycaemia.

D50 – Dextrose 50% in water. Administered in a 10cc syringe via IV.

EMD – Emergency Medical Dispatcher. Dispatcher who manages the various land-based units. Dispatches and manages crew requests on calls.

EMT – Emergency Medical Technician. USA term for persons responding and providing medical aid with an ambulance.

En route – Proceeding toward a call

Entonox Regulator – A demand regulator that is attached to an Entonox bottle. The patient must suck on the mouthpiece for the gas to be administered and is not continuous flow.

Epi – Epinephrine. Primary drug used to treat anaphylaxis.

Gauge – The size of the device being used. Same as is used to measure wire, etc. For example, 12-gauge, 20-gauge, etc.

GCS – Glasgow coma scale – A common neurological assessment scale used to determine the patient's conscious state. It assesses three primary areas: the patient's eye opening, speech and body motor control. The total best score is 15.

Glucogel – Oral glucose gel packs that are given to diabetic patients suspected of having low blood sugar.

GSW – Gunshot wound

Head bed – A C-spine head stabilization device.

Hyperglycaemia – High blood sugar. Normally above 15mmol blood sugar.

Hypoglycaemia – Low blood sugar, Normally below 4.0mmol blood sugar.

IM – Intramuscular – An injection at a right angle to the skin with a needle that is normally at least 25-gauge and 1 ½ inch long for an adult. It is designed to enter the muscular area of the body for faster absorption of medications than other types of through-the-skin injections.

ITT – Infant Transport Paramedic. Two-year program specifically designed for infant assessment. PCP may enter the program if they qualify. Completion of the program is intensive and challenging.

IV – Intravenous. Normally a solution of Normal Saline (Nacl) or Dextrose in 10% water (D10w).

IV catheter – An over the needle device that, after puncturing the skin, is inserted into a vein. The plastic catheter is forced into the vein with the needle used as a guide. After insertion, the needle is completely removed, leaving only the plastic catheter in the vein. The IV tubing or lock is then attached to give access to the vein for administration of medications or fluids as needed.

IV Line – The line that connects to the IV solution bag that delivers the fluid to the patient.

IV Pole – A small, telescopic pole that is attached to the side of the cot. It is extended to hang IV fluids to allow continued administration of fluids while moving the patient on the cot.

Kilo – A shift pattern where the paramedics carry a pager, are not in uniform until they respond to the ambulance station where they are given a minimum four-hour call-out. The remainder of the time they receive $2.00 per hour to carry the pager for the duration of the shift call-out that is twelve hours long.

Landmark – to identify the site and location on the chest prior to compressing for CPR

Lateral – When a job posting comes up and the successful applicant moves to that new station.

LOC – Level of Consciousness – A term used to describe the patient's level of consciousness as compared to normal.

MCI – Multi-casualty Incident. Any time the number of patients outnumbers the resources on scene capable of managing them, requiring a triage approach to patient care and more resources to be sent to the scene.

Mechanism of injury – The type of force or act on the body that caused the injury. For example, a fall off a ladder from 10 feet onto concrete caused a fractured leg. The mechanism of injury is the force of the fall applied to the leg, which caused the injury.

Medic – Medical assistant with the Canadian Armed Forces. They can be deployed in a hospital, field unit, or ship.

Meds – Medications

Naloxone – A drug that is an opiate antagonist. Used to reverse the effects of an opiate overdose, typically from heroin or Fentanyl.

Narcan – Naloxone

O2 – Oxygen

O2 Regulator – Device attached to an O2 tank or Entonox tank to lower the pressure of the tank in the O2 cylinder and provide an adjustable flow rate to administer in litres per minute.

O2 Tank – Pressurized tank that is filled to 2000psi with medical oxygen.

On Car Practicum – The time a paramedic student rides with an ambulance crew to be evaluated by a preceptor.

OPA – Oropharyngeal Airway – A curved plastic device with a channel that allows air to pass through it. They are colour-coded for size depending on the size of the patients jaw size. Yellow and Red are typically used for adult patients. OPAs are used for unconscious patients to help maintain a patent airway, or when using a BVM to ventilate a patient.

OTC – Over the counter. Refers to drugs available without a prescription.

P1 Course – Paramedic 1 course. Level of training in British Columbia before PCP became a national standard.

Pads – Defibrillator pads that are attached to the AED.

Papa car – A single-person paramedic response unit.

Paramedic – An emergency responder who is trained in emergency medicine to respond to emergency situations normally in an ambulance. Their role is to assess, treat and transport ill or injured persons to a hospital or higher level of medical care. Their scope of practice is dependent on the level of license they hold. They are licensed by an independent body outside of the employer and are responsible to maintain their license level as required by that licensing body. Their duties may require them to work out of helicopters, fixed wing aircraft, boats, bicycles, gators, or on foot, to gain access to or transport patients. They are authorized to use various medications and equipment to treat their patients that is provided by their employer.

Patent – Intact and functional

PCP – Primary Care Paramedic. Eight-month program, including practicums both on ambulance and in hospital. Paramedic that has basic level skills. They are trained to assess and make transport decisions based on patient presentation. They can administer a limited number of drugs, such as: Nitro spray, Epinephrine, Narcan, Gravol, Glucagon, TXA, Glucogel, and Benadryl. They are trained in AED, powered suction, KED extrication device, SAGAR traction splint, CPAP, and administration of IV therapy, including, NaCL, and D10W.

PE – Pulmonary embolism

Portable – A small radio that clips to a belt or is placed in a radio holster with a clip mic used for two-way communication when away from the Ambulance.

Pre-Alert – When a call is received by the 911 operator, the call taker sends the call to an ambulance crew to reduce response time. The call taker may still be getting details on the call as the crew begins its response.

Preceptor – A Paramedic who provides on car practicum, evaluation, and sign-off of Paramedic students prior to their final licensing exam.

Pt – Patient

Pulse Ox – Electronic device used to measure the Spo2 of the body and pulse rate with a finger probe placed over the nailbed. A LED light is used to measure the Spo2. Patients who are cold or have poor distal perfusion may give erroneous low readings. Nail polish should be removed, or the probe placed sideways to obtain an accurate reading.

Quarters – The ambulance station where the crew works out of, has bays for the ambulances, sleeping rooms, TV, cooking facilities, etc.

RCMP – Royal Canadian Mounted Police

SAR TECH – Search and Rescue Technician. Specially trained Canadian military personnel whose primary role is that of search and rescue. They are trained to be advanced medics, parachute, hoist from helicopters, and as Scuba divers and mountain climbers. They operate out of fixed or rotary aircraft.

SOB – Shortness of breath

SPO2 – Saturation percentage of oxygen in the body. Less than 90% is considered dangerous. Patients are typically treated with oxygen when below 95%. Normal is 98-100%.

St. John Ambulance – A volunteer organization that is paramilitary in nature. Members wear uniforms, conduct drill, and form up for parade and inspection. They are trained in basic and sometimes advanced first aid. They provide voluntary free first aid coverage for various public events.

Stretcher – A specialized stretcher, that is capable of multi-level height. Has four wheels, and locks secure into the back of the ambulance prior to transport.

Superintendent – Manager above a supervisor who is not part of the union.

Supervisor – Supervisor who is still part of the union. Normally works on the road in a single unit response vehicle that assists in dealing with issues and responding to calls when needed. The supervisor typically works solo.

Syncope – Fainting

Telfa – A thin, non-adherent dressing, often placed over a wound that has blood or body fluid seeping. Due to its smooth non-adherent material, the dressing will not typically adhere to the wound as normal gauze dressings would.

Trismus – Lock Jaw, often seen in patients who are unconscious, making opening the airway to insert an OPA or tracheal intubation tube impossible without sedating the patient to relax the jaw muscles.

Tutsi – Ethnic group located in Rwanda, Africa.

TXA – Tranexamic acid. Drug administered IV to assist in helping the body stop internal hemorrhage.

What is the process to become a Paramedic in BC?

Becoming a Paramedic in BC has changed over the years. When I was hired back in the fall of 2002, the ambulance service hired a person with a Class 4 driver's license, criminal record check and an Industrial First Aid certificate. You would be course loaded onto a part-time program — when one became available — that would take a year to complete. During this time, you could work at non-urban stations as a paramedic with your Industrial First Aid Certificate. I was given no emergency driver training at all. I still remember the first time I activated the emergency lights and siren, on the way to a call. I had no idea what all the siren tones were or how they could be used to help warn drivers. We would show up to a call with an ambulance, in uniform, and were no more trained than the first aid attendant working at the local logging camp or other industrial site. Fortunately for me my background as a medic in the military, St. John Ambulance, and the Coast Guard made the medical side of things much easier.

Today, fortunately, things are different. Every paramedic has to complete the 8-month program (including practicum and licensing) before working on an ambulance. The standards of care have increased dramatically, especially in remote communities.

The process to become a full-time paramedic has not changed though. It is a very long process and involves years of working part-time. Unlike the police or fire service, where you apply go through their application process, are hired and trained, and start a full-time career, doing that as a paramedic in BC is simply impossible.

Although every situation is different for each person, essentially once you are hired you are offered an area to apply for. Depending on vacancies at each station you will get a choice to pick one that you would find most suitable. The reality is that it will be a significant distance from your home unless you just happen to live in the town you are applying for. Many paramedics have to travel five hours to reach their new part-time station. I would say the average is three hours, but it may include ferry travel, which adds to the commute. You are required to be available for a minimum of eight shifts per month to maintain your seniority. This is important, as your seniority will dictate how fast you can lateral to another (hopefully closer) station. Once the primary station you are attached to uses up your availability, you are permitted to be available to work in urban areas such as the Vancouver post and pick up full paid shifts. If you only put in eight shifts available at your primary station, you may not get any left to work at other stations. If you put in 100%, you will get a lot of secondary work. Many remote stations have a relatively low call volume: 250-350 calls per year or sometimes less.

The pay is also dismal. When you arrive at your station for your start time, you are often on a 'kilo' car that is a call-out ambulance. You receive a whopping $2/hr. pager pay for the shift duration. If you get a call-out during that twelve hours you receive four hours at your rate of pay, typically about $20/hr. Most unit chiefs try to schedule you for back-to-back kilo shifts so you only have to make one or two trips to your paper station, so you can pick up work in the urban areas. I remember more than once staying three shifts in a row and not getting one call-out. The pager pay did not even pay for the travel. When working a 'kilo' car you are not required to stay at the station, nor stay in uniform. The idea behind the kilo car conception is that local living paramedics carry a pager, stay at home or in the area and are available to respond to a call-out, very similar to paid volunteer fire departments. The problem is that there are never enough local people interested or willing to work as a local paramedic. When new people are hired, in order to eventually work closer to where they live, they put up with the commute as well as the possibility of not getting paid enough to cover the travel or food to eventually get a full-time spot in the future.

After five years or so of jumping from station to station you eventually get enough seniority to apply for a full-time irreg spot. An irreg position is an irregular scheduled paramedic that works full-time, gets all the benefits, but does not have a permanent station to work out of. Normally what happens is you are pre-scheduled two blocks at predetermined stations normally not the same one. For the other two blocks you will often get called a few days before each one. So, essentially, you are a nomad, as you bounce from one station to another each block. Facebook is normally used to do shift swaps with other paramedics, so you can work closer to home or have a station of preference. Normally you have to work three to four years as an irreg paramedic before you finally get a reg spot. Very often this reg spot is located at least an hour or more drive from home, often much farther than you would like. It is not until you get a reg spot that you can lateral to other full-time stations. Sometimes you can get lucky and lateral in the next three months, other times you might have to wait up to a year. I was lucky that when I got my first reg spot it was not a popular station, but it was in Burnaby and I had a route that allowed me to avoid the Port Mann toll bridge, saving money on commuting. I was able to lateral to a station closer to home eight months later that was only 40 minutes from home and had no toll bridges.

Becoming a full-time reg paramedic takes on average ten years. So, when people ask me if I would recommend it, I often pause as I have a flashback of the time it takes. When people ask me if I like/love my job, I answer 'yes'; virtually all the paramedics I know do not go through that long arduous process for the money. There is no glory in being a paramedic. It seems that the local fire departments are able to maintain that image and we fall into the background.

What are the wages of a Paramedic in BC?

At the time of writing this book a full-time PCP paramedic will earn $32/hour on average, plus benefits. We have not had a wage increase in ten years and are below the cost of living increase scale.

Comparatively an RN makes $40 on average and by nine years makes $50/hour, a transit bus driver makes $29, and a garbage truck driver makes $28. I can bet that those other jobs do not take ten years to become full-time. Vancouver Police officers make $97,776/year, base salary. Vancouver fire fighters make over $100,000/year, base; this is more than critical care flight paramedics.

What is it like driving 'Code 3'?

When I started working as a Paramedic, driving 'Code 3' with the lights and siren wailing was exciting, and an adrenaline rush. Having the law give you the right to exceed the speed limit, and go against traffic control signs and lights, is something only an emergency driver is given. Part of the rush was the risk involved. Driving Code 3 is dangerous for both the vehicle responding and the public. Every year, ambulances, police, and fire trucks are involved in accidents when they are responding to or sitting at the scene of an accident or call. As paramedics, we normally start driving Code 3 in more rural areas with less traffic and few traffic control devices; more often, we travel down highways to get to an accident or rural address.

Working in busy urban areas is another story. Buildings bounce the siren sounds, so the direction of the emergency vehicle is difficult for some people to detect. Due to the often-heavy traffic, multiple lights at intersections, multiple lanes, and virtually sound-proof vehicles, civilians often do not hear us, even when we are directly behind them. The ambulances are equipped with high intensity strobes lights, but even with all of this we have to be extremely diligent to ensure that vehicles are stopping before we proceed past intersections.

Driving Code 3 puts everyone in possible danger: traffic does not always respond properly, people panic or stop directly in front of us, and some drivers block us in intersections at green lights! There is also the risk that accidents can happen when we think an intersection is clear and a car zooms through, hitting an ambulance. At times, we can sit trying to enter an intersection with our lights and sirens on, alternating tones and cars pass by sometimes completely oblivious to our presence. I often refer to people being in their 'zone' and completely clued out to things around them. This always amazes me, no matter how years I have driven 'Code 3.'

Life around the station

This section is about some of the things that happened around some of the ambulance stations I have worked. My full-time station at the time of writing this book was a very dynamic place to work. There were lots of ambulances and shifts with both regular and part-time paramedics working out of the station, with various shift start times to off-set the calls during higher call-volume times.

Washing the Ambulance

Washing the ambulances inside and out is part of our duties. Some crews are a bit lazy and don't pay much attention to it, knowing others will take care of it. Just human nature, or, perhaps, just a (lack of) work ethic. I personally enjoy working out of a clean ambulance. Depending on call volumes I make it my routine on my first dayshift to wash the outside and sanitize the inside prior to our first call. I also believe that showing up in a clean sparkling ambulance is a presentation of professionalism; that, and how our uniforms are presented goes a long way in the public perception of how we are viewed as health care professionals.

Platoon dinners

We had a paramedic who was like Martha Stewart. She would always bring in yummy baked goods: cakes, cookies etc. She was also the one who would spearhead a monthly platoon dinner at the station. Normally she would bring up the idea when there were a few crews around and suggest a date and possible theme, such as Mexican or Italian. A list would be made up with who is bringing what. We would normally have a lead of at least two weeks before the dinner.

The dinners were always planned on our split night which was our first night shift or third shift of the block. Some people would arrive a bit early to prep or get their dish ready to eat. The oven would be turned on and often the counter stops were littered with various crock pots and dry foods. Some items were placed in the fridge to be eaten later in the shift if we had a lot of extra food. Every theme dinner was a feast; everyone had a great time, and the food was fantastic. Bragging photos were always posted on Facebook so other paramedics could see. I always have fond memories of the camaraderie of bringing food in, sharing, and experiencing it together. Many times, crews would get calls and have to leave before eating, but plates of food were always put aside so if they happened to be out of our area for a few hours there would be food waiting for them in the fridge. When everyone had seconds, we would often bring some over to the ER staff at the hospital next to the station to share some of our creations.

Stories from around the station

Nude beaches

One day I arrived at my full-time station for a night shift. As I came into the day room, a few other crew members were standing around having a discussion about something and, within a few moments, I realized that the topic was again one of those unique topics that seem to cultivate themselves into a rather intense discussion; in this case, there was a humorous undertone. The crews were very intently talking about nude beaches and walking topless in public. Surprisingly, the variance of opinions was diverse. As I listened to the various positions on this subject I thought to myself, 'will people believe we talk about this at our station?'

Squatty potty

On another day, I walked in to hear a very qualified discussion on squatty pottys. I had no idea what they were, so after a few minutes I decided to ask the leader of the discussion (Jervis) what exactly they were.

I said, grinning: "What exactly is a squatty potty?"

Jervis turned to me, with a surprised look on his face and very directly replied: "You don't know what a squatty potty is?"

I said: "No, I actually don't."

Jervis shaking his head replied: "It's a small stool that you place under your feet when you are on the toilet. It is proven to make you poop better. You see, we are not supposed to poo seated, we are meant to poop squatting, but with technological innovations they invented the toilet. I use one all the time and it's great!"

I am sure I looked at him with a look of disbelief on my face, though I was smiling. Here he was articulating very intensely how to take a better poop on the toilet and that they have actually invented something to assist in that.

I said: "Well, sounds ridiculous to me. So, what do you do when you are here — not have a crap?" laughing now.

Jervis replied: "Well, Luc, I obviously just go anyway. I'm just saying it's a great invention and scientifically proven."

I said: "OK, well, I have nothing further to say on this, thanks for explaining it."

Jervis replied; "No problem Luc" He then turned to the others: "... As I was saying..."

At this point I left the room, smiling and chuckling at the conversations that happen at work.

Death Donuts

I remember the first time I came into the station and saw a box of Tim Hortons donuts on the dining table. At first, I didn't think much of it. I took a peek inside and noticed they were all chocolate. I found this a bit odd, as most times anyone buys donuts, they buy a variety to appeal to different tastes.

I commented: "Somebody likes chocolate donuts."

My partner looked at me and with a smile said: "Those are death donuts."

I am sure I had a puzzled look on my face when I replied: "Death donuts?"

My partner said with a very visual and dramatic expression: "You have never heard of death donuts!!?" "Where have you been?" he said, laughing now.

I had just been stationed at this station as my new regular post. Though I had worked out of this station before when I was part-time and Irreg, I had never heard of "death donuts."

Someone else in the station spoke up: "You have to buy death donuts when you lose someone during a cardiac arrest."

I replied, still puzzled: "So you fail to save someone and because of that you buy chocolate donuts?"

A new person spoke up who had also been sitting it the common room: "Yup! And you buy Timbits if you lose a child."

At this point, as I processed this new information I realized how morbid we were collectively as a group. I didn't ask at the time but considered that buying "death donuts" was to either make us all feel better about the death or as a punishment for not saving someone. I don't eat a lot of donuts and never did have one that day.

Some time later, I would see donuts arrive at the station, and sometimes crews would apologize for them not being all chocolate.

One day when the ALS crew bought donuts I said: "I guess you guys have to buy them often as when you show up and work the call they cannot be saved often."

One of the reg ACP, with his strong English accent, said: "No, it is the 1st crew on scene that is responsible for the death donuts if they die."

I replied: "Oh, why is that?"

He replied: "That's just the way it is, and always has been."

I processed this and in the coming months saw many boxes of donuts on the table. Fortunately, I almost never saw Timbits. The days did come where my partner and I had to buy death donuts as well. So, our station was known for our "death donuts"; this was not something other stations did and was unique to our station.

I take cream in my coffee

One day I stopped for a coffee at the local Tim Hortons. I am not a personal fan of their coffee and prefer Starbucks or other places that offer a richer, full-bodied taste. Coffee is important to me as I find I need it to keep myself going when I am lacking sleep!

On this particular day when I went in for a coffee, they had come out with a new "dark roast" and I wanted to try it. I normally take my coffee with just cream, however I have noticed that most times when I have asked for cream the pre-set measurement is too much so I will modify the amount and try to use the lingo that the establishment uses to make it easier. I used to order my medium coffee with a small cream to make that adjustment. On a previous visit, the staff member told me to just say "½ cream," and on the register screen it would display "½ cream" so it made sense. So that's what I did on this particular day.

I walked up to the counter, and the female staff member said: "Can I take your order?"

I replied: "Yes, I will have a medium coffee with ½ cream."

She looked at her screen, began touching various buttons. Afterwards she looked up and said: "Would you like anything else?"

I replied: "No, just the coffee, thanks."

She said: "It will be ready for you over there," motioning to the small pick-up counter.

As I waited, my partner, Tim, was waiting for his order as well.

A few moments later, the woman placed my coffee on the pick-up table and said: "Here is your coffee sir"

I replied: "Thanks."

I grabbed the coffee, flipped up the plastic lid tab, and took a sip: I almost spat it out! It was awful. I peeled off the lid and looked at the coffee, and it was as white as a sheet of paper. I was a bit puzzled now, wondering how much cream she put in the cup.

Smiling, Tim looked at me, and said: "Is there something wrong with your coffee?"

I said: "Well, yes, there is a lot of cream in this coffee, take a look!"

Tim looked into my cup and replied "Yeah, I'd say," with a grin.

I looked for the woman who made my coffee, but she was busy behind the counter. After a few moments, she looked in my direction.

I said: "Excuse me, how much cream did you put in my coffee?"

She looked at me and said: "½ cream."

It took a moment to process this, and, still confused, I decided to ask for clarification.

I said: "½ cream?"

She said very matter-of-factly, while using her fingers on a cup to show ½ cream was in the cup and replied: "Yes ½ cream."

I am not sure if the disbelief in what I heard was as evident as I thought, but Tim was virtually busting out laughing at this point, trying to contain himself.

I said to her rather intensely at this point: "Well, I wanted ½ the amount of cream you normally give for a medium not ½ a cup of cream with my coffee!"

She looked at me somewhat annoyed and said: "OK, I will get you anther one — so you want ½ of a shot of cream then?"

I said, "Yes, thanks," still a bit in disbelief that she had actually filled a cup ½ full of cream, then added coffee.

I was given the new coffee, peered inside to make sure it looked like it should, and took a small sip. Yes, this one was good. Tim laughed all the way on our walk to the Ambulance.

"You know Luc," he said, "that would only happen to you."

I replied with sarcasm: "Thanks."

My journey to become a Paramedic

My interest in becoming a paramedic went way back to my youth. It all started with the TV show *Emergency*. This was a 70s show about two EMT paramedics that worked out of a fire hall and responded to medical calls. They would stabilize the patient, often calling Rampart hospital asking for medical orders based on a patient's presentation. These EMTs were not able to operate independently but had to consult with an emergency physician located at the local hospital before administration of medications or doing procedures. In 1973 at the young age of 6, I found this fascinating. I would often play games pretending I was a paramedic and even used props of plastic bags and tubing to simulate starting IV lines on patients. This is where it all began.

As I grew older I continued to be interested in helping people and learning about first aid and medical care. In 1982 at the age of 15 I joined St. John Ambulance, a voluntary world-wide organization with a para-military structure that devotes itself to providing free first aid coverage for local events. I became very involved and was fascinated by the military structure and uniforms. I remember being very proud to wear the uniform and represent the organization.

A year later I also joined the local SAR (Search and Rescue Team); it was not until I left the team seven years later that it was realized that I was not supposed to be permitted to join the team at the young age of 16, as I was supposed to be 19 years of age. I was very active on the search and rescue team, by volunteering for virtually every search, and attending all of the training sessions. I even became a qualified military air spotter with 442 Search and Rescue Squadron out of Comox, BC. Participating in various live and practice searches I quickly attained over 50 flight hours in a Labrador SAR helicopter, and 30 hours in a Buffalo. During my time on the team, I moved into the positions of Equipment Officer, Training Officer, and Vice-president; the year I left the team, I was voted into the position of President, which I turned down as I was leaving for the military. I joined the military to become a SAR tech (search and rescue technician). It looked like the best job in the world, being a rescue guy: parachuting, rescue diving, mountain climbing, and being an advanced medic; I could not imagine a more exciting and rewarding career.

Back to the medical side of things: In 1986 at the age of 19, I completed and took my first major recognized first aid course, back then known as Industrial First Aid. This was the standard industry first aid course that was recognized in the province of BC. If you wanted to work as a first aid attendant in BC, you had to have this course. It was two weeks long and involved a lot of self-study and practical scenarios. At the end you had to be tested by a workers' compensation examiner; this included a 100-question multiple-choice written exam and practical. I passed with solid marks and was awarded a "C" Certificate (70% minimum). At the time there were four levels based on your practical and written marks: C, B, A, and AA. On your first course you can only get a C level no matter what your marks were. If you were successful in achieving a higher level on future courses, it would extend the recertification date up to four years for level A. I completed the course the following year and earned a level A (minimum of 90% on written and practical exams). Even paramedics working on an ambulance had to hold an industrial first aid certificate at this time. I began riding third on the local ambulances to gain some insight into the career.

As I participated in St. John Ambulance, I became a first aid/CPR instructor. I was very shy when I was younger and being involved with St. John Ambulance and SAR pushed me out of my comfort zones. I joined the military as Med-A (medical assistant) in June of 1990, with my goal to apply for SAR Tech in four years. At that time a soldier had to wait a minimum of four years to apply to re-muster to the SAR tech trade. After spending six years of regular (full-time) service with the military, and with various personal circumstances, I was not willing to stay in longer to attain the dream SAR Tech trade, even though I was sent an invitation to re-apply the year I was getting out of the military. I had made it as close as less than 10 from the selection of the last course. Since they only run one SAR tech course year and the second year I applied the entire course was cancelled for the year, I was definitely unlucky. My second three-year contract was up in 1996 and I took my honourable release from the military. I had a very interesting and exciting 6 years while working as a Medic. Most of my time, I was attached to a field Ambulance Unit in Petawawa Ontario. During my service, I was trained to drive a multitude of vehicles including an APC (armored personnel carrier), and even a snow machine. I went to Lahr, Germany in 1991, and Rwanda, Africa in 1994 on a Humanitarian mission ('Operation Passage'), shortly after the genocide of 800,000 Tutsis. I was in the Airborne jump section, part of the Airborne Battle group, which was itself part of the elite Airborne Regiment composed of the three commandos at the time. I was a pharmacy stores technician, and spent a total of two years working in various hospitals in different roles.

Upon release from the military in 1996, I worked a few jobs and attended college. In January 2000, I was hired by the Canadian Coast Guard Hovercraft Unit in Richmond BC, beside the Vancouver International airport. I began training as a Rescue Specialist and Rescue Diver.

In November of 2002, I was hired as a part-time Paramedic and began working in a station in the town of Lytton, BC. I started my year-long part-time P1 course in January 2003, while I continued to work full-time at the Coast Guard as a Rescue Specialist Diver. As I progressed through the course I was able to pick up shifts in Chilliwack, BC as it was not considered urban. I completed my P1 course in January 2004, and was able to work in the city of Vancouver. I wanted to gain as much experience as I could, so working in part-time call-out stations was a slow way of gaining experience. I picked up as many shifts as possible in between working my full-time job as a Rescue Specialist and fulfilling my obligations of 1 or 2 trips to my paper station. I spent 2 ½ years in Lytton, then did a lateral move to Boston Bar, BC for a short six months. I lateraled from there to Whistler, BC and stayed for two years until I was able to lateral to the town I was living in, Abbotsford, BC. I worked part-time in Abbotsford (4-6 shifts per month) until I decided to work full-time as a paramedic in February 2012. While working Irreg for approximately 3 ½ years, I became a paramedic preceptor and trauma instructor. I finally was successful in obtaining a full-time reg spot in July 2015 at a station in Burnaby, BC. I was now able to lateral to other full-time stations depending on seniority and availability. I successfully lateraled to a station in Surrey, BC in March 2016; this was the highest call volume station in all of BC.

About the Author

Luciano Nisi immigrated from Italy to Canada as a young child. His passion for writing this book came about because of a desire to share his experiences as a Paramedic. His interest in being a medic dates to his full-time service with the Canadian Military. For six years he served as an Airborne Medic parachuting from aircraft with his medical bag, assault rifle and rucksack, taking care of the soldiers, he served with. He is also the author of *Crossing the Line: How to Cross a land border Stress Free*, and *Trail Ready: How to Pack and Prepare for Hiking Emergencies*. He is currently writing his fourth book: a memoir of his life as a soldier. When he is not writing, he enjoys flying airplanes, photography, and hiking in the backcountry. He currently lives in Abbotsford, BC.